THE PERSISTENT OBSERVER'S
GUIDE TO
WINE

*How to enjoy the best
and skip the rest*

by J. P. Bary

Neon Press

A division of PdB Partners, Incorporated

Greenwich, Connecticut

D1112944

www.neon-press.com

Where trademarks, servicemarks or other proprietary rights may exist initial capitalization has been used to designate names. However, no attempt has been made to specifically designate as trademarks or servicemarks all terms in which proprietary rights may exist. The inclusion, exclusion or definition of a word or . term is not intended to affect, or express any judgment on the viability or legal status of any proprietary right claimed in that word or term.

The information contained in this book is true and complete to the best of our knowledge, but any recommendations that might be expressed or implied are not guaranteed by the author or the publisher, each of which disclaim any liability in connection with the use of such information.

© 2012 by Paul de Bary.

FIRST EDITION

Bary, J.P.

The Persistent Observer's Guide to Wine: *How to enjoy the best and skip the rest.*

Summary: "An engaging introduction to wine that concentrates on the reader as much as the wine, pointing out the most common pitfalls and sources of confusion as it proceeds step-by–step through the essential skills everyone needs in order to select, serve and store wine properly and pair it with various foods and occasions successfully."—Provided by publisher.

ISBN 978-0-9858400-4-4
ISBN 978-0-9858400-2-0 (ePub version)
ISBN 978-0-9858400-3-7 (Mobi version)

Library of Congress Control Number: 2013900044

PRINTED IN THE UNITED STATES OF AMERICA

December 2012

To my parents, who taught us to investigate things, search for the true path and keep ever close the vision of Paradise.

To our kind "Uncle" Donald Keene, who first brought wine to our home.

To all my partners in wine, especially:

Vickie, Ned and John de Bary
Diana and Peter Samponaro
Leslie and Charles Rousell
Lin and Tracy Lavery
Gabrielle and Richard Bolton
Martha and Dominique de Anfrasio

Contents

Introduction

Making your way through the wine labyrinth isn't that difficult once you get your bearings, but most people lose their way after a few wrong turns. In my own early wanderings, I often found myself at the intersection between success and failure without knowing how I got there or which way to turn. Despite efforts to read the map, I ended up on long detours or in blind alleys repeatedly. Indeed, much of what I read seemed to have little relationship to the landscape I saw in front of me. So until I learned how to recognize the little signals that kept me from going around in circles, I stumbled along a twisted but well-worn path for many years.

It's not that I didn't learn quite a bit about wine during those rootless years. It's just that only a small fraction of what I learned was really useful. As I look back now on what helped me the most, the key guidelines I use today don't seem to be terribly complicated or hard to fathom. Just a few persistent mistakes and misconceptions kept me in the dark. I can't help wishing I'd figured them out earlier.

Part of what confused me was my assumption that a prodigious effort was required to truly understand wine. The task of becoming proficient always seemed daunting and somewhat mysterious. I was told I needed to improve my wine vocabulary, master the geographic subtleties of various wine regions and take detailed notes. But for me, wine was an easygoing companion. Why spoil a carefree relationship by taking it too seriously?

It was also too easy for me to believe I was picking up what I needed to know just by doing what came naturally. Supportive retailers treated me as a valued customer, less knowledgeable friends deferred to my judgments and occasionally a sommelier would compliment me on "a good choice." Deep down, however, I was often disappointed with the decisions I made and knew I wasn't getting it quite right. So I persisted in trying to learn more, though I sometimes wondered if I would ever have time to learn all I needed to know.

The books I've read about wine over the years could more than fill my modest wine cellar. Most were written by well-recognized experts. Some entertained me with stories, others featured clever layouts and graphics to help me visualize and memorize a host of details. Beautiful photos of vineyards, wineries and, of course, elegant people delightedly sampling the product inspired me and brought back pleasant memories of evenings when every drop of the lustrous liquid in my glass seemed precious. With the right wines meals tasted better, conversation flowed more easily and my life just took on a brighter glow. Yet those "right" wines seemed frustratingly difficult to find. It wasn't simply a matter of paying more or choosing wines the experts had rated highly. Despite what I was learning, I still experienced disappointment as often as success.

As I tried to learn more about wine, I attended tastings led by professionals. Yet there was a wide gap between what the professionals said and what I experienced. I could sometimes pick out different tastes when they suggested them, but could almost never pick them out on my own. I even became suspicious (rightly so in a few cases) that what I was being told was simply a put-on. After all, most of my friends couldn't connect what they read or heard about the taste of a wine to what they actually experienced. Were we all the victims of an elaborate hoax, or just missing some elusive wine-tasting gene?

For a long time, I learned more than I needed to know, yet not enough to make a real difference. So many things influenced the experience: food, friends, storage, service, even the shape and temperature of the glass. It was all pretty bewildering. But gradually I realized that what was helping me most wasn't so much what I had learned about wine as what I was learning about the mistakes I kept making.

These mistakes weren't things I read about in books. I had to figure them out for myself. Yet, as I learned how to avoid them, my success began to increase steadily. And as I shared the lessons I'd learned with others I found I wasn't the only one making these mistakes. I still wasn't a great expert on wine, but I was becoming an expert on wine mistakes, and could help others figure out what confused them, so they could enjoy their wines more as well.

I think I can now appreciate why it's so difficult for wine experts to write a useful introductory guide for ordinary consumers. It's easy for beginners to get lost in the details as they first attempt to find the patterns woven deep in the fabric of wine's rich tapestry, but as one learns to recognize them these patterns begin to seem obvious. Since the details no longer obscure the basics, it's easy to assume that everyone else understands them too. Meanwhile, the hard-won skills you've developed become so instinctive that you employ them unconsciously.

So it occurred to me that it might be useful to have a wine guide written by someone who hasn't become too much of an expert. I seem to be at a sweet spot in the progression from neophyte to connoisseur: far enough along to understand what the experts are trying to say, but still able to connect with what confuses the ordinary consumer. If I can't soar high enough to command the entire landscape, I've at least scratched the dirt long enough to learn the difference between a kernel of truth and a poisonous pest.

I don't intend to cover the same well-trodden ground as other wine books. This isn't a slimmed-down wine encyclopedia. It doesn't describe a single wine region or drop the names of legendary wines I've sampled with famous producers. There are no rules about how to taste or serve wine and no diagrams segmenting the tongue or showing the interactions between flavor elements in food and wine. Nor are there any defined terms you need to master before you can understand what I'm saying.

What I'd like to share with you is something different. I've asked the muse to help me keep the focus of this book on you and how you experience wine. Rather than classifying and presenting wines in the abstract, I want to help you develop an understanding of them as you drink them, without having to memorize anything. I'd like to give you a better context for your wine experiences by revealing the natural processes and human interventions at work behind the scenes, so you can sort through all the confusing details by yourself and make better choices without the need of expert assistance. You'll learn how to think for yourself about wine, so you can overcome whatever challenges you in a way that's best suited to your own particular needs.

In this book I describe serious mistakes that millions of people make every day—mistakes I've made many times myself. Once I describe them to you, you'll see why they're so easy to make and why they're such persistent barriers to a deeper understanding of wine. Then I'll help you remove those barriers so you can get closer to wine as a living, breathing organism and become intimately familiar with its personalities and moods. You'll learn to pick out the special qualities that different grape varieties contribute to a wine and see how they're modified by climate and manipulated by winemakers. You'll see how each glass communicates with you in its own way and be able to build a deeper rapport with the wines you love best. You'll also get better at spotting the troublemakers early, so you can keep them at a distance or maybe even make them behave.

In a few short lessons, I'll show you how to avoid disappointment and be energized, rather than intimidated, by the choices you have to make. Then surprises will be something you look for and part of what makes wine more exciting. You'll come to understand why, in the world of wine, complexity isn't a curse; it's a compliment.

Many books promise to simplify wine, but it's complicated for good reasons. Oversimplification ignores wine's greatest virtue and leaves you oblivious to its most unpredictable and thrilling pleasures. Yet the devil isn't in the details, either. While a good book can help make the arduous process of learning the many fine points of wine a bit easier, knowing all those details won't protect you from most of the frustrating mistakes and misconceptions that ruin your wine experiences. By learning more about those common mistakes and misconceptions, you'll master the art of choosing and enjoying wines much more quickly than you will by learning all the fine points. In this book, I'll clear away the biggest obstacles that keep you from enjoying wine at its best, so your wine experiences will become more rewarding with each chapter and you'll find more pleasure than you ever expected in each new glass you drink.

Being Tasteless

Start with the end result

To disregard the taste of a wine is to ignore its reason to exist. Wine may nourish us, quench our thirst and give a pleasant lift to our spirits, but it gets our attention with its taste. If that doesn't appeal to us, we'll drink something else.

It's curious, then, that so many people pay so little attention to the taste of the wines they drink, and it's disconcerting to think of all the good wine and money being wasted as a result. Every day, in restaurants and retail shops, people ignore advice about taste or are just oblivious to the issue. How often, for example, do we see a group at a restaurant proudly order one of the most expensive wines on the list and ask that it be served right away? Then they'll order spicy appetizers and salads drenched with vinegar or topped with palate-smothering cheeses—dishes that destroy the ability of anyone to distinguish between the expensive wine and ordinary plonk. After quickly polishing off the expensive bottle, the group will then order wines better suited to the appetizers they've just finished, which inevitably arrive just in time to overwhelm the taste of courses that would have been better complemented by the expensive wine.

Does it make sense to buy an expensive wine and then proceed with the rest of the meal as if its taste didn't matter? Not if the taste is what you're paying extra for.

Taste Blindness

When asked to think about it, most people agree that taste is the most important quality in a wine. Yet it isn't usually the first thing they think of when choosing a wine. In fact, it's often the last thing they think of. Why is that?

In my case, it was mainly because I didn't make the right connection between taste and value. Overwhelmed by the noticeable disparity in the prices of the many different wines available to me, my first concern was with whether I was getting my money's worth. I felt I needed to understand "quality," and that was something I had a very hard time putting my finger on.

Over the years, I've found many others who've shared this concern, and the wine industry seems to appreciate just how widespread it is. Most efforts to sell wine involve some variation on the value proposition. One is that a wine is a great bargain. Examples of this range from a breathless "I know this is expensive, but it's really priceless!" to a cynical "I know this tastes bad, but at least you won't spend a lot of money on it!"

Another way that wine marketers address our concern over value is by trying to persuade us that the inherent quality of a good wine justifies its higher price. This approach usually has more substance behind it, but their pitches can include everything from sly misdirection to transparent fraud. At the lower end of the market, pedestrian wines may be dressed up to look like their nobler cousins, while at high-end auctions fake bottles of legendary wines are passed off by counterfeiters secure in the knowledge that the wines aren't likely to be consumed immediately, if ever.

Even if you filter out commercially motivated pitches and clever chatter from the more earnest references to wine quality, there are many competing views of what quality is. Wine professionals and connoisseurs usually have strong and well-informed opinions on the subject, but they often disagree, which doesn't exactly help those of us who like to keep things simple. But as I've come to understand these disagreements, I've found them to be largely a matter of taste. They agree that a higher-quality wine should taste better, just not about what tastes better.

It's not surprising, then, that most people are as confused as I was about wine quality, even when they tell me it's the first thing they think of when they choose a wine. But even though they'll readily confess to being a bit uncertain about what quality is, they're still sure they want it. Problem is, since it's a matter of taste, there's no fixed and immutable standard of quality in a wine. In fact, understanding your own sense of taste is the only place to start if you want to get good value when you choose a wine.

Lost in Taste

For many years I had only the vaguest idea of what a particular wine might taste like when I saw it in a shop or on a restaurant wine list. Even though I could taste wines when I drank them, I had difficulty recalling the taste when choosing a wine later. I could easily identify with the couple standing in front of a wine shop in a *New Yorker* cartoon. One says: "I think we've had that wine before, but I can't remember whether it was good or bad!"

My taste-blind wine selections continued long after I began attending wine tastings, reading tasting notes and visiting tasting rooms at various wineries. I gradually became familiar with the taste of a few of the more affordable wines I drank regularly, but when I wanted to step up and buy a better bottle for a special occasion or order from a restaurant wine list, I had little idea what the wines available for me to choose from would taste like. The only thing I could say for sure was that 99.9 percent of the wines in the world wouldn't taste much like the ones I was familiar with. Sometimes, even the taste of those changed.

I wasn't entirely alone in my confusion. Sometimes, as I shared a glass with friends, I would ask what they thought the wine tasted like. Perhaps they would murmur something about "body" or "fruitiness," but for the most part, even when they had a glass in hand, the only thing they were sure it tasted like was, well…wine! Did it have to be any more complicated than orange juice or Coca-Cola?

The answer should be obvious, of course, but it took me a while to realize that what makes wine different is precisely the wide variety of tastes it can have. Wine producers compete for your attention by trying to distinguish their wine, not only from other beverages, but also from other wines. This gives you a better range of selections for wine than you normally have with drinks such as tea or coffee, or even soft drinks, juices, beer or liquor.

All that variety offers us better choices, but it can also lead to confusion and disappointment. Without a clear sense of what a particular wine will taste like, it's hard to know how well it will suit your needs or your pocketbook.

The Problem with Prices

While inexpensive bulk wines can be quite tolerable in the right circumstances, most of us tire of them if we have to drink them too often. They're also not likely to be the kind of wines we'd consider for a special occasion or to enhance the experience of a specially prepared meal. When we set out to purchase a more expensive wine, however, it's difficult to know what it will taste like, since it's unlikely to be a wine we can afford to drink every day. In fact, the minute we move up the price scale from bulk wines, we enter a very competitive arena where variations in taste and price abound. This is where the action is, where we can find the quirky and the overlooked, and where it's easy to stumble on something unexpected. Lamentably, as cost increases, so does the risk of making mistakes.

We're accustomed to thinking that a higher price should be a protection against disappointment, however. Simple economics also suggests that the price of a wine should be dictated by the relationship between its supply and the demand for it. We're tempted to apply this simplistically and assume that demand should be greatest for the wines that taste best and that higher-priced wines should taste better than cheaper ones.

But taste is a relative matter. The French say: *"Chacun à son goût!"*; the English: *"There's no accounting for taste,"* in ancient Rome, *"De gustibus non disputandum est!"* A wine won't necessarily appeal to you just because it appeals to many others, and there are all sorts of other things that affect the taste of a wine: its age, the temperature you drink it at, the food you eat it with…even the mood you're in when you drink it. Great wines transcend many of these factors, but none can transcend them all.

A compounding problem is that there are only so many wines the average consumer can learn to recognize in a lifetime. For reasons we'll get into later, wines that achieve celebrity status tend to be produced in limited quantities compared to their renown. While the laws of supply and demand may work handsomely for them, they don't necessarily result in equivalent prices for many other lesser known but equally worthy wines. Even Adam Smith was concerned about the price inefficiencies of wine.

Despite these complexities, however, the global wine distri-bution system does a remarkable job of satisfying the tastes and needs of millions of happy wine drinkers who every day embrace the challenge of sorting through all that variety. You might find it a bit intimidating at first, but it's really not difficult to master the skills that make the process fun rather than fearsome. The most important skill needed is one you already have: the ability to taste.

To get the most out of any glass of wine, you need to be able to taste it properly and have a sense of what you like or dislike about it. If you know why a wine pleases you, you'll be better able to find others like it. More important, if you understand what you don't like about a wine, you're in a better position to judge whether it's something you want to avoid in the future or a good wine you're just dinking under the wrong circumstances.

Your Natural Ability to Taste

The first step toward understanding any wine is quite simply to taste it and ask yourself what you first notice. Although the answer should come naturally, it can be difficult to put a finger on it at first, since we're naturally influenced by what we've been told about the taste of wine in the past and feel obliged to come up with something similar. But trying to remember what it is you're supposed to be noticing at the same time you're trying to notice it can be a pretty challenging task. Fortunately, it's unnecessary.

Next time you start to drink wine, put aside whatever you've been told about the art and science of wine tasting. Don't try to focus on the "attack," the "mid-palate," the "aftertaste" or any exotic flavor. Just take a moment and concentrate on what stands out in your overall impression. You might experience a sense of heat, a tingle or a feeling that your tongue is getting rough. You might be a bit overwhelmed by sweetness or bitterness or notice a pronounced flavor that's familiar to you. Just take your time and get comfortable with the fact that you can pick up quite a bit of information on your own.

For too many of the years I spent aimlessly wandering in the wine wilderness, I was hindered as much as helped by well-meaning wine aficionados eager to share with me what they tasted in a wine. I could almost always find whatever they suggested to me if I concentrated on it hard enough, but it usually wasn't something I'd tasted before they suggested it to me.

Once I became comfortable identifying tastes for myself, the tables suddenly reversed and others almost always found the same things I did. Like the golden bough emerging from the Sybil's breast, this was a precious passport to a deeper understanding of wine. With my newly gained confidence, my own sense of taste emerged from the shadows and the impressions of others could be put in their proper context. I could pass through the ivory gates and begin to chart my own course.

Initially, my newfound confidence made me eager to offer advice to beginners, just the way others had given advice to me. Each time I suggested a taste and a glint of recognition came from across the table, I thought I was helping another lost soul along the road to wine appreciation. What I failed to realize was that the most important difference between us was not a vast store of wine knowledge, but simply my confidence in the ability to taste for myself.

Instead of telling inexperienced tasters what *I* was finding in the wine, I should have been asking them what *they* were finding and helping them appreciate what discerning tasters they already were. We all use our sense of taste every day and can easily tell if something tastes good or not. To taste wine well, we don't need to change that, just understand it better and learn how not to interfere with it.

Almost always, when someone suggests a taste to you, you'll find what was suggested, but if it wasn't what you noticed yourself, it won't be so easy to find it again. So instead of trying to find something exotic, like a "*soupçon* of asparagus," or poetic, like "silkiness," just begin your exploration of wine by concentrating on tastes you feel are either overwhelming or noticeably missing. It's more important to understand what *you experience*, and connect that with what *other people say*, than it is to focus on something you've heard and try to find it.

As soon as you start to concentrate on your own taste, you'll find it easier to understand what you like and dislike. Then you'll naturally want to learn more about the taste of wine so you can enjoy it even more by avoiding wines that aren't pleasing to your own palate and choosing those that are. Since you are the only person with the knowledge that enables you to do that, it doesn't work to substitute the judgment of others. Their judgments can be interesting, but they'll help you only if you have a judgment of your own to compare them to.

How to Start Tasting

The process of learning to taste wine is a bit like learning to field a ball. You have to start by simply doing it. At first, the ball coming toward you can seem a bit frightening, but as you become more familiar with the various incoming trajectories your reactions change from instinctive alarm to instinctive response. Gradually, as your confidence builds, you take pride in your ability to anticipate an unusual bounce and learn to handle what originally seemed out of reach with grace and aplomb.

I hate the idea of an "educated palate," because for me each glass of wine is an education. It does help, however, to learn to recognize the basic taste elements in wine, just as it helps to learn to recognize the trajectories of a ball. This is much easier when you're actively involved and building on what you already know. Whether you've learned to conceptualize it or not, you know what you taste. Rather than learning to find something in a wine you don't already recognize, it's better to learn to recognize what others call the things you already find.

Once you stop trying to remember what it is that you're *supposed* to taste and just concentrate on what you *actually* taste, your first reaction is likely to be a sense that a wine has too much or too little of something. Does it seem a bit too sweet or too dry; too thin or too heavy; too rough or missing that bit of kick you enjoy when you finish it? These are clues to your sense of taste and how it relates to wine.

When you concentrate on what you yourself taste, it's natural to think about what you enjoy most or least, which might or might not be what you notice first. You may find it interesting to pay attention to the last thing you notice about the taste of the wine. Since your first impression is likely to be influenced by residual tastes in your mouth, different qualities can emerge as you drink more of it. What you notice last is likely to be quite different from what you notice first and might even be what you like best.

A Sense of Balance

The tastes you notice for yourself, particularly those you like or dislike, are things you can easily remember and look for the next time you try a glass of wine. As you start to identify things you find too much or too little of in a wine, you'll also start to build a natural understanding of the term "balance" and you'll instinctively realize that it's a relative term rather than a fixed ideal.

The concept of balance in a wine is often talked about, but many people find it confusing. This shouldn't happen, because most people can learn to appreciate balance fairly easily. The mystery isn't so much how to recognize it as what makes it happen.

Many references to balance suggest that it's simply a matter of offsetting sweetness with sourness (which most wine writers refer to as acidity) on some sort of linear scale. Simply equalizing the levels of each of these qualities doesn't create balance, however. Rather, it's a matter of letting all the most desirable qualities of a wine emerge by making sure that nothing else dominates the taste. So, for example, a level of sweetness that might distract from the delicate flavors of a light white wine could blend almost imperceptibly into the bolder flavors of a full-bodied red wine.

Many wines are prized for attributes, such as aromatics, dryness or weight that complement a particular food or style of cuisine. Like a mechanic balancing the wheels on an automobile, a winemaker will add or subtract a little something here or there to help the wine show off these attributes. When you learn about balance by picking up on what's missing or overwhelming in a wine, you appreciate intuitively that there are too many elements involved to measure balance in any precise linear way. Rather, balance involves a kind of restraint; it's a quality that makes all the ingredients in a wine blend harmoniously into something indefinable, where the whole is equal to more than the sum of the parts.

Wine writers often refer to this in younger or more full-bodied wines as "character" and in older or lighter wines as "finesse." There are other terms: "breed," "harmoniousness," "elegance." These don't need to be defined; you know them when you taste them. For you, balance will be a little bit different than for anyone else, but you shouldn't worry about whether you can taste it. If a wine seems one-dimensional and uninteresting, it's unbalanced; if there's something special going on and the wine seems to resonate and be evolving as you drink it, you're sensing balance. It's actually what makes a wine stand out and get noticed—what winemakers and critics spend most of their time looking for—yet we all can sense it quite naturally.

Let Go and Take Control

Once you connect with what seems harmonious to you, you've begun to develop a sense of your own unique way of tasting things. Don't be afraid to run with it. Taste is deeply entwined with our primitive instincts for survival and growth, and it can be a bit intimidating when you first experience the full extent of its capabilities. But this is only an affirmation of how well suited we are to take our unique place in the wild riot of life. Nothing smells as fragrant as a meadow, as fresh as a sea breeze. When we feel good, we say life is a bowl of cherries. Somehow, everyone knows just what we mean.

Whether we encounter it in a tended garden, a vast wilderness or the majesty of the night sky, we have a deep-seated ability to enjoy the sights, smells and tactile sensations nature offers. The natural world breaks down the remnants of unpleasantness and returns them to us as luxuriant new life. It is this world that the vine inhabits and pours forth in the taste of wine. With roots deep in the soil, it pulls up the elemental juices of the earth. Its leaves and tendrils stretch out to the warmth of the sun and stir in the scented air of the mountain valleys and maritime hillsides it inhabits.

With care and skill, winemakers can use the natural cycles of fermentation and gentle repose to concentrate, digest and refine the wild flavors that surround and permeate grapes as they struggle to survive and flourish. With any well-crafted wine, these tastes can be found in plentiful diversity and are constantly evolving and changing, even as they sit in the glass. No one can describe them all with perfect precision; it's actually quite an achievement just to be able to describe the few you're most likely to find.

Don't Always Believe What You Hear

When you have difficulty matching the taste of a wine to what you've been told about it, the reason is usually quite simple. Don't discount the possibility that what's been described simply isn't there. Although it's not unheard of, you're unlikely to find exotic tastes in inexpensive wines. Their tastes aren't the ones that wine writers wax poetic about, but that doesn't always prevent their marketers from using a little poetic license. A producer promoting a wine will understandably emphasize the tastes consumers are most likely to seek, even if these aren't the ones they're most likely to find.

Similarly, while some restaurants make an effort to familiarize their staff with the wines on their list, others concentrate on training them how to sell whatever is on it, regardless of whether they are familiar with it. One young fellow told me proudly how he had been trained to sell wine when he worked as a waiter. If he was asked what a wine tasted like, he was told to answer according to whether it was red, white or sparkling. If it was red, it had "soft fruit"; if it was white, it was "minerally"; and if it was sparkling, it was "toasty." When I asked him if that was what he tasted in the wines, he said he really wasn't much of a wine drinker, but found that little formula good enough to impress most people.

In my experience, people who can succinctly and effectively communicate what they taste in a wine are extremely rare. It's understandable that these writers can give proper attention only to a small fraction of the wine the world drinks each year and prefer to devote their attention to the world's greatest wines. Yet the greatest wines are the most difficult to describe adequately with words. You shouldn't let that keep you from enjoying them. Neither should you let the fact that no one will ever write about most of the wines you drink keep you from learning how to taste them.

Trust Your Own Good Taste

Even if you're a rank beginner, there isn't much you need to learn in order to get the best out of wine. What you need is just enough knowledge to keep you in your comfort zone and out of a disorienting trap. Then the idea that you don't exactly know what to expect will make each experience richer and more exiting, like trying a new delicacy being offered to you by an old friend or having a meal prepared by a great chef who delights in coming up with new and surprising tastes for you to enjoy.

To be able to keep yourself in your own wine comfort zone, you'll need to understand a wine's basic structure and how things like grape variety, climate, and winemaking style affect it. You'll also want to learn how to store your wines, serve them and drink them properly. The basics of each of these subjects are easy to understand and we'll take them up in turn. But the most fundamental skill you need to enjoy wine is the one you've been practicing since the day you were born. You don't need to learn how to taste wine the same way someone else does or become a walking wine encyclopedia in order to enjoy wine's natural and man-made wonders. Trust your own sense of taste and let it be your constant guide as we continue on our way.

Whenever you take a glass in hand, remember to concentrate on what you're tasting and experiencing yourself. Learning to understand which wines appeal to your personal preferences is the easiest way to maximize your drinking pleasure and become comfortable with the value you receive when you purchase wines. Concentrate on what you enjoy and you'll build that understanding on a solid foundation, one you'll be able to draw on readily and use confidently. Just don't forget that the most important aspect of taste is the overall impression it conveys and that the thrill of the unexpected is one of wine's predictable pleasures.

In the next few chapters we'll delve more deeply into the taste of wine and begin to pick apart its different elements. I'll show you why you can easily get confused by some of the things you hear about wine and you'll learn how to avoid the most common misconceptions and troublesome distractions that interfere with your understanding of the wines you drink. Then you'll be able to focus your natural wine-tasting ability on the things you enjoy most. Those won't be too hard to find or so easy to forget.

Taking Shortcuts

Enjoy the scenic route

People who are passionate about wine always remember that first transcendental moment: the exact time and place when an unfamiliar wine began to speak to them in a surprisingly intimate way. If it hasn't happened to you, it's something to look forward to.

It's almost never love at first sip. Often it's the last sip that does it. Suddenly, the thought that you might never taste this wine again seems devastating and you realize you've been taking it for granted. If you're lucky, your glass will be refilled and you can draw the wine close, savor its scent and revel in its intoxicating embrace, entering a state where everything else seems incidental because you're so intently focused on the wine. Time itself seems to slow down.

There's a message hidden in that special feeling. Our surrender to wine's slower rhythms is a necessary part of the experience. In order to enjoy the best of what it has to offer, we have to learn to make time for wine. But in the haste to reconnect with the transcendent moments, it's easy to lose sight of this. We try various shortcuts and end up getting lost, victims of ignorance and wine's special versions of divination, numerology and idolatry. All that's necessary to avoid these pitfalls, however, is an understanding that drinking almost any wine can be a deeply rewarding experience.

You have an innate capacity to take pleasure from wine, and learning how to take full advantage of it isn't as difficult as you might imagine. All you need is to incorporate a few simple steps into your wine-drinking routine and take the time to gradually absorb what you learn as a result. To do it most efficiently, though, you'll need to resist the temptation to take shortcuts, since they'll only slow you down. Most of them involve excluding from your consideration the very wines that will please you most. I know it's counterintuitive, but by taking your time and giving every wine its due, you'll actually develop your understanding of wine more quickly.

Shortsighted Shortcuts

Because there are so many wines and so many differences among them, it's natural to look for shortcuts to wine happiness: simple techniques to filter out all the wrong wines we might choose and leave us with only sure-fire winners. When people try to streamline the wine selection process, however, they have a tendency to oversimplify things, and that doesn't make their selections better, just quicker. Having a decided preference for very dry white wines doesn't mean there won't be times when a red wine or a sweet one will seem absolutely glorious. If the shortcuts we take simply narrow our choices, all we do is limit our options and keep ourselves from learning how to enjoy wine more, in different ways.

The notion that there's a simple way to find appealing wines more quickly isn't the only reason we're tempted to take shortcuts. Self-image and our troublesome vulnerability to peer pressure also play a part. In fact, the shortcuts we take usually reveal more about us than they do about wine. Being told that a connoisseur can find quality wines at inexpensive prices, a frugal person may be inclined to believe that only cheap wines are worth considering and judge the value of wines only in terms of price. Religiously ordering only the cheapest wines, a penny pincher will only waste money and could get better value drinking water.

The super-rich are at the other end of the spectrum, of course. They can afford to drink only the most expensive wine and, not surprisingly, there are quite a few people out there willing to sell it to them, whether it makes sense or not. It might be a horrible match for the food they've just ordered, but when Mr. and Mrs. Fitch choose the most expensive wine on the list, the sommelier is more likely to compliment than object, even though a higher price has much less to do with how suitable a wine will be than a host of other factors. True, food isn't the main event when you order wines made for a billionaire's palate, but it's hard to admire someone who substitutes flaunting of wealth for knowledge of wine.

Most of us are easily able to avoid these extremes, of course, but we're still hampered by certain preconceptions and limitations when it comes to understanding wine. That's why it's important to recognize some of the many other less easily recognized shortcuts that can tempt us, and understand why they don't work.

Why It Doesn't Work to Start at the Top

Art Buchwald, the legendry humorist and food and wine reviewer for the Paris edition of the *Herald Tribune* in the 1960s and '70s, once described his early efforts to pretend he was an expert on wine as "learning a few big names and throwing them around." We smile because he's making fun of himself and so many others.

Of course, name-dropping is as common and obnoxious in the wine business as it is anywhere else, but Buchwald ultimately became quite a connoisseur of wines, and I think he was trying to convey a more serious message through his humor. Many people assume it's easier to learn about wine from the top down than from the bottom up, so they shortcut the learning process by paying attention to only a few prestigious wines. Yet there is a world of difference between learning all the top names in wine and learning to understand wine. In fact, starting at the top is a bit like assuming that the best place to learn mountain climbing is on the summit of K-2 or Mount Everest. You're more likely to slip and fall than learn anything useful.

The greatest wines are the most difficult to understand because complexity and intangible nuances are among their most highly valued qualities. They would not be quite as special if they had only the attributes we expect to find in our everyday wines, nor should we expect to find in our everyday wines the attributes we value most in great wines. Everyday wines have a job to do, and we only become snobbish and superficial when we take what they do for granted. If all we learn about are the unique characteristics found in a few very expensive wines, we're learning about things that don't exist in most of the wines we drink on a regular basis. As the journeymen of the wine world, these more modest wines have their own individual talents: flavors, textures and other qualities that bring out the best in food and friends. These are talents we can put to good use on a daily basis.

I must confess that, at certain points in the earlier stages of my wine education, my desire to learn was propelled by something more than natural curiosity. Like Buchwald, I was anxious to appear in the know, especially to those I considered privileged to drink the world's most prestigious wines. Knowing a bit more about wine seemed to offer a bit of a toehold when I felt under social pressure. On those glittering occasions when I suddenly felt painfully less attractive and successful than everyone else, it was comforting to know a little more than others in the room with respect to at least one subject that was likely to be near at hand.

Looking back, I realize now that at least a few of those listening to me (probably the ones with the most encouraging smiles) actually knew much more about wine than I did, but were kind enough not to dampen my enthusiasm by pointing out my mistakes. Inevitably, I also ran into others who were playing the same game I was, knew some obscure fact about the subject I didn't and delighted in taking me down a peg. For a while, I foolishly tried to avoid this by doubling down; memorizing more and more about the wines from the most prestigious wine regions and producers, even though I wasn't likely to drink them very often.

Learning prestigious names and places did increase my familiarity with the leading wine regions and make me more knowledgeable about the leading wine producers. But there are hundreds of leading producers around the world. Each year they make new wines that are carefully scrutinized and rapidly snapped up by knowledgeable and affluent buyers. One could dedicate hours and hours to learning about them and only have the wherewithal to drink their wines a few times a year, if at all. Eventually, it became clear to me that keeping assiduous track of them was more trouble than it was worth.

I also wasted a great deal of effort by spending hours studying expert opinions about the most subtle and hard-to-understand nuances of wine long before I had an understanding of its basic structure. Since I couldn't really connect these with my own experiences, the only thing I learned was that the experts' opinions were better than mine. In the end, what I thought might be a shortcut into the ranks of the wine elite just left me with doubts about my own judgments, more dependent than ever on the opinions of others. In my haste to be hip, I accepted the opinion of anyone who was held out to me as an authority without testing it against my own experience. This slowed me down because I accepted as true much that was wrong and understood wrongly much that was true. I was simply out of my league.

Regional Myopia

Many people find it useful to concentrate on the wines of a particular region as they begin to build their knowledge of wine. This is a strategy I highly recommend, particularly when the region is one whose foods you find appealing, but it can work against you if you don't understand some of the hazards you can encounter along the way. Because it filters out all the wines from other regions, it seems like a shortcut, but you can delve so deeply into one region that you can't find the way out.

Europeans, especially those who live near world-renowned wine-producing regions, often think that they don't need to know anything about the wines produced in other parts of the world. Confident that France makes the best wines in the world, most French wine drinkers see no reason to learn about anything else, while other Europeans, happy with the wines produced at home and daunted by the sheer scope, diversity and cost of French wines, invent deficiencies in French wines they don't really have.

Even smaller regional biases play a part. The Bordelaise and Burgundians are each convinced they have inside access to the most sought-after wines in the world, so why should they look elsewhere? The gastronomes in Turin look down their noses at Chianti, while the Florentines hiss that most Barolos aren't worth the price. Provincialism won't prevent the lucky people in these areas from drinking good wine, of course, but it does leave them a bit narrow-minded.

A friend of mine travelling in Tuscany spent a few days in Siena, the heart of the region where Chianti Classico wines are made. He had developed a fondness for "Super-Tuscan" wines, which are made from different grape varieties than typical Chiantis. Since Super-Tuscans are made nearby, he was surprised to find none available in the restaurants or wine shops in Siena.

Montepulciano is another nearby wine-producing area in Tuscany. It's a little bit warmer than Siena, but the wines are made from a special clone of Sangiovese, the same principal grape variety used in Siena. As my friend was visiting a winery near Siena, his host asked where he was going next. He replied that he was gong to Montepulciano. Clearly offended, his host asked: *"Perché bere quelle spazzatura?"* ("Why would you drink that garbage?") Obviously, even though he made good wine himself, he had a rather narrow view of what it was.

All too often, as they master the nuances of a particular region, its disciples start to share the locals' biases against other wines. As a result, they needlessly ignore wines that might better match the foods readily available to them or the occasions most suitable to their own climate. The ability of great Clarets, Barolos or Chiantis, and even some Burgundies, to stand up to barbecue is a testament to their greatness…but a waste of their talents. There's a reason why Australians love their barbie with a simple Shiraz.

During the nineteenth and twentieth centuries, outmigration from Italy, China, India, the Middle East and Central America spread the tasty foods from these areas around the globe. As a result, our diets today aren't limited to the cuisine of a single region. So, if you begin your explorations with the wines of one area, understand the limitations you inherit with that strategy. Wines from Bordeaux aren't as easy to understand if you drink them with curried rice or sweet and sour pork.

As you find wines you like, be particularly alert for situations where they don't work for you. Unless they seem to enhance the foods you eat most often, be prepared to try different wines with these foods. As we'll see later, some common foods can be particularly tough on wines. Respecting the limitations of your favorite wines will help you enjoy them more, because you'll be less likely to force them out of their comfort zone. Situations where they don't provide the pleasure you normally expect could be a regular part of your lifestyle. Do them a favor and find a better match.

Flying Solo

With all the emphasis I placed on trusting your own taste in the last chapter, you might think the simplest way to avoid getting lost in the details would be to rigorously avoid taking advice from anyone else. In fact, when their initial experiences with wine advice leave them confused, many people simply try to make their way through the world of wine on the basis of what they can learn for themselves. After making little progress, however, they often simply lose interest in wine.

What's important to keep in mind about your own taste is that it's unique. Without understanding it, you won't be able to appreciate the limitations on someone else's ability to speak directly to your palate. You're also impressionable, so if you start to explore wine by looking for what others describe, you'll almost always find something, even if it's the wrong thing.

While simply relying on what others say isn't a shortcut to wine happiness, neither is going it on your own. Since the landscape of wine is too richly textured for you to discover all it has to offer on your own, you'll want to take advantage of the knowledge gathered by the millions who've traveled through it before. The most reliable way to build your wine knowledge therefore is to *start* with what you experience and *then* measure that against what others describe. They can help you avoid the bogs and briar patches and tell you where, with a little effort, you can find the spectacular vistas. Stubbornly following only your own sense of direction is likely to lead you into a dense thicket of endless taste-blind selections.

Relying on Your Retailer

It's often said that the best way to obtain good wines is to find and follow the recommendations of a good retailer. This is generally good advice, particularly if your wine buying is limited to holidays or a few occasions when you're entertaining at home. But it's not the best way to improve your knowledge of wine. To improve your knowledge of wine, you have to not only get good advice, but also understand why it's good.

As someone who works full time in the trade, your retailer should know quite a bit about wine and should also be able to predict your needs and tastes. (Retailers who can't anticipate the needs and wishes of their customers don't stay in business long.) A good retailer will sense the level of your interest in wine and try to use it for mutual advantage. By learning about the wines you like and the foods you eat, a retailer can help you make more successful choices and establish a frame of reference for what a good wine experience should be.

The best retailers have a knack for hospitality and can often anticipate your needs without much discussion. But you still need to think for yourself. If you always rely on someone else to choose your wine, how will you get to know what you're drinking and why? When you rely on your retailer so much that you can't make a good choice when you're in a restaurant, you've traded off what should be some of your most enjoyable wine experiences for a bit of everyday convenience. Rather than just taking recommendations from your retailer, try to make sure you understand the reasons for these recommendations and take advantage of the opportunity to learn a bit more about wine.

Don't assume that all retailers have the same high standards, however. In larger shops, some of the clerks might not be all that knowledgeable and might not be prepared to admit that to a customer. Smaller shops might not have that many customers with a serious interest in wine, so the management may need to rely more heavily on liquor or beer sales. That will make it difficult for them to recommend much beyond the few wines they stock. You should also be alert to the fact that many retailers tend to specialize in one type of wine or another, usually the ones they like best themselves.

Before you put your trust in a retailer, make sure you've found a person who's both knowledgeable and sincerely interested in helping you get the most from the wines you buy. Look for someone who tells you about the taste of the wines and asks about your likes and needs before making a recommendation. Be wary of anyone who loads you up with big names and doesn't ask about your dietary preferences and entertaining habits. It takes a bit of time to build a good relationship with a retailer, but the time you invest will pay handsome dividends for both of you.

Rule Rigidity

Taste isn't an ideal subject for regulation. It's intensely personal, subjective and susceptible to the fickle dictates of fashion. Yet we have a deep-seated urge to make order out of chaos. Faced with what appear to be confusing choices, we reach out for guidance and look for direction. Without direction, we may be tempted simply to follow the crowd. But a leaderless crowd can get ugly. Give it direction and we feel safer following it. So either way, we end up following someone else's rules, either consciously or unconsciously.

The effort to fashion appropriate guidelines for wine consumers is as difficult and controversial as any rulemaking process. Civilized people, moreover, rarely dedicate themselves to learning all the fine points, exceptions and loopholes in any set of rules, relying on a general understanding and their own common sense to keep them out of trouble. Sophisticated wine consumers treat wine rules the same way. When someone tries to apply the rules too rigidly, they're more likely to be amused or become annoyed than to pay attention.

As you develop your interest in wine, you'll read more about it and hear more about it from friends who share your interest, as well as from retailers and other professionals. In the process, you'll inevitably be introduced to numerous rules about how wine should be made, sold, stored, served and consumed. Some are well known and others less so, but most can be helpful as long as you understand their limitations and treat them more as guidelines than rigid requirements.

Most of the rules about wine are useful. If they aren't, they get discarded. But the popular understanding of the rules is often imperfect and even the rules you receive from a trusted source can reflect misunderstandings, regional or commercial biases, or outdated preconceptions. Often, a rule that is perfectly sensible in one context takes on a life of its own and is misapplied in other contexts.

It's the nature of regulation that what seems perfectly obvious and reasonable at first blush ends up being much too simplistic and confining to work in the real world. For example, it might seem beyond dispute that grapes shouldn't be harvested too early. What could be simpler than developing a guideline for each variety of grape? But in Germany and elsewhere it's common practice to make different styles of wine from the same grape variety. So, for example, Riesling can be used to make a fairly dry wine labeled Kabinett, a sweeter Spätlese or a very sweet wine labeled Auslese, which is made from late-harvested grapes. Obviously, what's way too early for an Auslese could be just fine for a Spätlese or Kabinett.

It's also obvious that any rule about when to harvest grapes has to take into account all the subtle differences in microclimate that exist between one plot of land and another. As a result, in areas where there are regulations about when to harvest, they are often hotly contested or circumvented, particularly if they are too rigid. Alternatively, regulations can be so broad as to have little effect. Most rules about wine are like this, whether formalized as regulations or not. It's important to look behind them, try to understand the reasons they exist and test them against your own experience.

I spoke once with a fellow who had received a bottle of wine from a legendary château in the Bordeaux region of France as a gift. Although he wasn't much of a wine buff, the name of the wine was so well known that he felt compelled to treat it with respect. So he carefully tucked the bottle away in a quiet corner of his closet and began to research the wine. He learned that the wine was from an excellent year and gathered up many details about the region it came from, the legendary family whose name was on the label and the soil in the vineyard.

He also read several reviews of the wine. They all rated the wine very highly, but gave slightly different recommendations about when to drink it, most of which seemed a bit too distant. So he took the earliest one, added a year for safety, rounded off to his next birthday and set that as the target date for consumption. He figured he might not drink the wine at its peak, but he'd be close enough.

In the course of his research, he came to realize that the closet he was storing the wine in wasn't at the perfect temperature, so he moved the wine into the back of his refrigerator to make sure it wasn't overheated. Then, as the appointed date neared, he began to research how to serve the wine and what to eat with it.

On the Internet, he found instructions about how to decant wines. They recommended that "big" red wines be opened at least an hour before they are served. Since one of the reviews he had read said the wine was full-bodied, he figured that would apply.

He also found a review of a tasting where the wine had been served paired with ravioli of Argentinean shrimp and wild mushrooms in a foie gras-truffle sauce. He loved shrimp and the pairing was chosen by rock-star sommeliers working with celebrity chefs, so he didn't think he could go wrong. Conveniently, the review reported that a consensus of the gourmets at the tasting was that the sauce was a bit spicy for the wine, so he figured he could do fine without it and designed his own recipe for a ravioli made from shrimp, wild mushrooms and cheese. Both he and his invited guests apparently enjoyed it immensely.

I could tell that he had told his story about the birthday dinner with the legendary bottle of wine often. Yet when I asked what the wine tasted like, the fellow seemed a bit surprised, as if no one had asked him that question before.

"It was nice," he said, "although I couldn't really taste any of the things they mentioned in the reviews." Then he began to voice some slight reservations: "Some of my guests thought I should have served it with meat, but I knew that was an outdated rule. One of them also thought I shouldn't have stored the wine in the refrigerator. What do you think?"

I reassured him a bit and asked how the wine compared to the ones he was used to drinking. He confessed that it didn't taste as flavorful as he had expected, but extolled the "wonderfully flowery and delicious" fragrance of the wine when he had first poured it into the carafe. The fragrance didn't seem quite so obvious when he served the wine over an hour later, however.

All in all, what had made the occasion special for him was the excitement the illustrious wine had generated among his friends, who all assured him how delicious it was before they left, despite any reservations they may have voiced earlier. Even though he didn't actually remember much about the taste of the wine, it had still been the focal point of a memorable evening.

By any standard, one would have to consider the wine a major contributor to the success of this intimate birthday party. The few nagging doubts weren't so much about the wine as about whether the host had stored it or served it properly. It's curious though that the humble ravioli seems to have pleased everyone as much as, or maybe more than, the wine. One wonders whether, if they hadn't been so worried about appreciating it properly, they all would have enjoyed the wine as much as the ravioli—or maybe they wouldn't have bothered to mention it at all.

It was a bit unsettling to sense the reservations that this fellow still harbored about his universally acclaimed wine after all the effort he'd made to consume it "properly." Almost every preparation he made was dictated by some wine rule: The wine was put away until it was deemed ready to drink. Great effort was made to keep it cool during most of the time it was stored and to let it "breathe" before it was served. He consulted an oracle on the question of food pairing and did the best he could to follow its advice, although, had he been able to speak directly to the gods, they undoubtedly would have told him: "Don't try this at home!"

He tried to follow the rules, but didn't really understand what they were for. So in the end, they may have hurt more than they helped. The rule just says store your wine at 55°F (13°C) and drinking windows assume that the rule will be followed. Learning the rule doesn't teach you how quickly the flavors might be cooked out of the wine in a warm closet or how much its maturation might be slowed down in a refrigerator. Without a place to keep the wine at that magic temperature, all he could do was wing it and worry.

Clearly, it's best to understand the reason behind a rule before you try to apply it, and be suspicious of any rule that's categorical. You should never think less of a wine you enjoy because it seems to violate a rule; almost every wine breaks some rule. Above all, don't expect to find pleasure in following the rules; look for pleasure in the wine and let the rules help you find it. If a rule doesn't help you enjoy wine more, put down the rule and drink the wine.

The Golden Rule

Each temple of wine has its own oracles. From time to time, a sage local worshipers turn to for advice emerges as a prophet whose teachings are inscribed in stone and treated by some as commandments. You may find it helpful to follow these commandments. Just remember that wine doesn't read them and be cautious about applying them too rigidly.

I've found only one rule about wine to be universally applicable. Before you learn any others, master this: *For every rule about wine, there is at least one exception, usually more.*

When I first thought of trying to organize what I was learning about wine by making a coherent set of notes, it seemed reasonable that I could sift through all the rules, discard the outdated and elucidate the confusing. I imagined I could iron out any inconsistencies among those that remained, boiling the rules down to a limited, but highly effective, set of strictures. This would be the ultimate shortcut to wine success.

I searched diligently for such a simple set of rules, but didn't find it. Without all the exceptions, what's left is a short list of oversimplifications. Try to include them, however, and the rulebook becomes unwieldy and, inevitably, incomplete. The gift of a few fail-safe rules is a shortcut that no one can or should provide you with. Wine's subtlety and diversity, and its ever-unfolding mysteries, make every rule a moving target, while its unexpected pleasures are always the most delightful.

For many people, debunking various rules is part of the fun of drinking wine. They delight in learning all the wine rules because they know there will be exceptions and enjoy the sport of turning the rules inside out. At some point, you may have fun doing this as well, but you'll want to have fun enjoying your wine first. To do that, you need time to thoroughly understand the basics before you become confused by too many rules and exceptions. Struggling with rules that don't always work isn't the best way to begin building a solid base of wine knowledge; neither is learning exceptions to rules you don't understand.

Taking Your Time

It doesn't require a crash course on all the rules and their many exceptions to learn to make the best use of wine's abundant gifts. All it requires is that you take a bit of time and learn to gather your thoughts and spot cues you might otherwise miss. Once you take the time to pick up these cues, you'll be surprised how quickly you'll progress.

One of the first things you'll notice, if you take the time, is how much taste there can be in a single sip of wine. Simply let it sit in your mouth for a while, and you should be able to tell if a wine is going to really deliver the goods. The next time you have a clear palate and a few moments to concentrate on the wine you're drinking, take a little swig and squeeze it back slowly until it covers your entire tongue. Let it sit in your mouth and warm up for a while before you swallow it. Then give yourself some time for the overall impression to sink in.

If the wine gives you pleasure, it will immediately be apparent, whether you know a hundred rules about wine or none at all. You'll feel a bit uneasy that you might have rushed through the whole glass without appreciating how much pleasure it could give. If, on the other hand, the wine leaves you dissatisfied, you won't look forward to the prospect of drinking the rest of it. Lo and behold, just by taking a little time, you've become a connoisseur!

Most people have an innate ability to judge good wines from bad, even if they can't explain why. I love to serve a great wine without fanfare and just sit back. Sooner rather than later, people will start to say: "Is there any more of that wine?" I probably should have warned them not to drink it so quickly, but I love their uncoached affirmation that I've chosen well. It also answers a question I'm often asked: "What do I need to know to appreciate a great wine?" The answer, as by now you know, is "nothing special."

When you take time to concentrate on their taste, you'll notice many different flavors, textures and other qualities in the wines you drink. Because they're numerous and change from wine to wine, it takes time to develop a thorough understanding of them. This isn't a reason to be intimidated by wine as much as a reason to be more adventuresome in drinking it. It's this endless variety that ensures you will never tire of it. But when you're first learning to identify the different qualities that wines can exhibit, it helps to keep things simple. You only need to understand how to identify a few basic characteristics in order to learn how to select the wines you'll enjoy most. Then you can begin to master the more subtle nuances simply by drinking those wines.

Start with the Fundamentals

It's easier to pick out wine's finer points once you've mastered the basics. But the basics often escape our notice because they seem obvious. It's only after you've developed a conscious awareness of the fundamentals of wine that you can appreciate how important they are.

One of the most fundamental characteristics of wine is the interplay between sweet and sour tastes, and it's fairly easy to develop your awareness of this. We've all added sugar to various drinks, such as coffee or tea, to sweeten them to our taste, so it's relatively easy for us to sense the degree of sweetness in a wine and judge whether it appeals to us or not. In some white wines, particularly sparkling ones and those lightest in color, there is hardly any sense of sweetness, because almost all the sugar in the grapes was converted into alcohol during the winemaking process. Other white wines, particularly those with a deep golden color and syrupy texture, can be among the sweetest things you will ever taste. Red wines are more likely to stay in the middle range but can also vary in sweetness.

Sweetness is easy to sense because it relentlessly insinuates itself into our consciousness. The tiny residuum of sweetness in a bone-dry wine tugs at our taste until it secures recognition. In sweeter wines, it floods over us and sinks in, leaving a persistent imprint as the wine washes away. The sweetness of sugar softens the wine and can dull our sense of taste if overdone, but the sourness of acidity enlivens it by mounting a fierce but fleeting assault. Each wine's unique mix of acids rushes at us with a lively battery of weapons and provokes a dramatic response, summoning our digestive juices and animating the appetite. This is why it serves as a natural counterbalance to sweetness.

This dynamic interplay between sweet and sour is apparent the moment we pause to contemplate the taste of a wine and it receives as much quiet attention from wine professionals as the subtleties of flavor that often take center stage when the wine is discussed. Like the harmonic convergences of a musical scale, there is no single center of equipoise between sweet and sour, and what appeals to you can change depending on other qualities in the wine. It can also depend on your mood and how you feel about the stylistic preferences of the winemaker. This is why the experience of tasting wine is so intensely personal, and why you need to connect with it for yourself before you reach out for the opinions of others.

There's a difference between simply learning things about wine and building an understanding of it from personal experience. It doesn't take any special training to appreciate the basic differences in sweetness among wines or to sense the sour assault of its overall acidity. But by simply taking the time to observe the interplay between them, you can develop a deep understanding of the most fundamental forces at work within a wine. You'll learn that when they blend harmoniously, it's easier to find other exciting qualities in a wine and, when they don't, it's useless to try. How can you start to build a framework for comparing one wine to the next without taking the time to experience how its sweet and sour qualities interact?

Just taking a bit more time with each glass you drink will help you develop a deeper relationship with wine and increase your understanding of its basic dynamics. When you sit down with a bottle, each glass will be a bit more mature than the last. You may be able to observe the wine as it emerges from its youth and gains maturity right in front of you. Your relationship with the wine may mature as well, and qualities that seemed attractive at first may become boring or be overshadowed by others you hardly noticed. Just by giving it a little attention, you'll develop a better relationship with the wine and begin to sense instinctively what you can expect from it.

The Instant Critic

Once you begin to trust your wine instincts, your understanding is likely to advance more rapidly than you expect. You may even have to resist the temptation to declare victory prematurely. It's easy to learn to recognize just a few traits, notice how much of a difference they make and begin to think you've learned enough. But don't become complacent. The greater prize comes when you remain alive to the endless variety wine offers and keep giving it the opportunity to show you new tricks.

Though you can learn a lot from the first sip, it's a terrible injustice to judge a wine by your first impression. Like well-trained athletes who sense opponents' moves from tiny cues, many wine professionals can lift a glass, take a short swig and expound at length on the qualities of the wine. They could probably spend twenty minutes talking about the wine before they even taste it, and what they say wouldn't be much different from what they say after they taste it. When they do this well, it's natural to admire them, but you don't need to emulate their speedy pronouncements about the wines they taste. Remember that they've been trained to take maximum advantage of what they see and smell in a wine before it ever touches their lips. They've also had years of experience putting wines in context and learning how to verbalize what they experience—years you should be looking forward to.

Now that you've learned to take a few extra moments with your wine, become more aware of its taste as you drink it, track it as it evolves, pick up its resonant balance or awkward imbalance and thrill to its unique and subtle nuances, there is no reason for you to be in a hurry to sound like an expert. If you like a wine, pay it a compliment; if you don't (and saying so isn't impolite), say that too. You'll be surprised how many folks there are out there who can relate to what you're saying. So, here you are, you haven't even finished two chapters, and you're already making judgments about wine and chatting amiably about them with kindred spirits. As you can see, it doesn't take long to get comfortable with wine if you take your time.

One thing you can learn from the experts is this: people who know wine best are least likely to express categorical opinions about it. They've learned that tastes differ and that any glass of wine can be full of surprises, so they're respectful of the various perspectives of others. What they're looking for is a fresh and spontaneous insight, not a rote recitation of facts from someone else's compendium. You can recognize the true expert by the bemused smile that flashes when someone says something stupid about wine. So if you aspire to be recognized as truly knowledgeable about wine, just be humble and concentrate on what you know best—how the wine tastes to you.

Enjoy the Whole Experience

Richard Feynman, the physicist and Nobel laureate, had a prodigious intellect and a fertile imagination and also knew a great deal about wine. He gave a lecture series for non-science students that was recorded and later published by Cal Tech in the book *Five Easy Pieces*. At the end of one lecture, he asked his students to reflect on a poet who once said: "The whole universe is in a glass of wine." To Feynman it was the stuff of physics, the twisting liquid venting gaseous molecules, the reflections in the glass:

> What strange array of chemicals are in the wine? How did they come to be? There are the ferments, the enzymes, the substrates, and the products. There in wine is found the great generalization of life: all life is fermentation.

For all his scientific musings, however, Feynman was able to appreciate the beauty of what could not be analyzed. He understood that an excessive focus on details can lead to simplistic characterizations and reminds us not to forget the main event:

> If our small minds, for some convenience, divide this glass of wine, this universe into parts—physics, biology, geology, astronomy, psychology, and so on—remember that nature does not know it! So let us put it all back together, not forgetting ultimately what it's for. Let it give us one more final pleasure: drink it and forget it all!

There is neither satisfaction nor glory in being a wine dilettante. If you don't take the time to experience wines fully and respect their subtle differences, your understanding will only be superficial and the facts you learn of limited value. Knowing where a particular château is located or who owns it is interesting, but it doesn't help you distinguish the taste of red wine from white. There's no point knowing the great vintage years in each of the world's premier wine regions if you don't understand what it tells you about when to drink the wines.

As we progress through the next few chapters, you'll learn much more about the taste of wine and its various components. As you concentrate on these components, just remember to take a little extra time to ground yourself in the overall taste of the wines you're drinking. Collecting facts can be useful, but every glass of wine contains a sea of them. Those most important to you will reveal themselves only if you give them time to rise to the surface. Once they do, they'll have a personal meaning and leave an impression you can draw on in the future without memorizing anything. Shortcuts will only limit your options and cut you off from wine's most valuable quality, its rich variety. Take time to connect with what you enjoy. Build pleasant memories and understanding what to do with them will come naturally.

Wine is hard to understand, but easy to love. Like a bosom companion, it can be transparent yet remain an enigma; share itself freely while only slowly revealing its mysteries. It asks nothing from us except that we spend a bit of time with it after a busy day. No one can, or should, simplify that experience for you. If they do, you'll never have time to develop the deeply rewarding relationship with wine you both deserve.

Tripping on Your Tongue

Understanding your palate

Introductions to wine often devote considerable attention to explaining your palate, or, more prosaically, your tongue. Sometimes, there's a diagram dividing the tongue into sections named after different taste buds with complicated names like foliate, fungiform, filiform and circumvallate. It will show the lower edges of the front and side as sensitive to sweetness and saltiness and the back to bitterness. The area in the very middle of the tongue is sometimes identified as sensitive to "weight" or "touch." What's left, a fairly broad portion along the top edges, is identified as sensitive to sourness.

With a little practice people can use an understanding of their taste buds to begin to differentiate the degrees of sweetness, sourness, bitterness and saltiness in the wines they drink, but I don't really see anyone telling the ordinary wine drinker what to do with that information. So I have my doubts about how useful it is when you're first learning to taste wine.

No one taking a sip of wine actually experiences its taste in the neatly defined way the taste-bud diagram suggests. In fact, all the different taste buds are distributed throughout the tongue. If you touch it with your finger, you actually might find the tip and edges more sensitive to touch than the middle. Put some salt on the tip and salt taste buds will react, not sweet ones. There are even taste buds that aren't on the diagram, so it can be a bit misleading. What it shows is simply where the taste buds that sense certain taste elements are concentrated, not precisely where a particular taste is experienced.

Did you say, "Now I get it!" when you read the beginning of this chapter because you didn't know what I meant by sweet and sour in the first two chapters? Do you normally think of the difference between sour and bitter in terms of where you taste them? Do you need to concentrate on the sides of your tongue to know how salty something is? Of course not!

I can't really think of any situation in which wine experts actually use the segmentation of the tongue to describe the taste of a wine, unless perhaps you consider the term "fruit forward" to have something to do with fungiform taste buds, which is unlikely. I'm sure it's been tried, but no one differentiates the taste of wines according formulas that quantify the amount of sweet, sour, bitter and salty ingredients. Instead, they just jump right into describing wine flavors by analogies to fruits, spices and other foods. I even know of one introductory wine book where an engaging and otherwise knowledgeable wine writer claims that there's no salt taste in wine. So, you see, you can have a whole set of taste buds missing and still have a promising future in the wine business!

The Problem with Microanalysis

Now that you've seen how much taste there is in a glass of wine when you take some time with it, you may be itching to plunge in and find all the exotic tastes wine writers wax so poetic about. I'm going to help you do that, but microanalysis of your tongue, or even of the wines you drink, isn't the best place to start. That's because you need to understand the basic structure of wine, and place things in their proper context, in order for the more exotic elements to emerge from the mix.

When I was first introduced to wine tasting, I found the alcohol level in wine the easiest quality to judge. Higher alcohol wines generate a sense of "heat" in the mouth. By comparing my guesses to the alcohol content listed on the labels, I was able to gradually make more and more accurate assessments of alcohol content. Once I became fairly proficient, I used my newfound ability as something of a parlor trick.

One evening, as I was trying to impress some friends, one of the younger women in the group asked a pertinent question: "Are the alcohol listings on the labels often wrong?" Blushing, I had to admit that I didn't know and assumed that the labels were usually correct. Fortunately, she didn't ask why on earth I had been so proud to be able to extract from the wine the one piece of information everyone could readily obtain just by looking at the label!

My foray into alcohol levels may have been a bit embarrassing, but it taught me several things. The first was that, by paying even haphazard and sporadic attention to a single element of taste, I was able to learn to recognize fairly subtle differences in the wines I was drinking. Another was that excessive attention to the microdetails of taste could lead to "paralysis by analysis" and become a distracting impediment to my overall enjoyment of wine.

Eventually, I learned to make proper use of my ability to assess alcohol levels as a key factor in what's commonly referred to as "body." Definitions of this term vary all over the lot. (For fun someday, try comparing the definitions of tasting terms in various wine books.) Some treat it as simply a question of how much alcohol there is in a wine, while others concentrate on what counteracts the astringency from higher alcohol levels. Still others equate it with "weight," which is another tasting term that wine professionals use more because they can sense it than define it.

It can be interesting to speculate about the dynamics of body, but I've never found anyone, even a rank beginner, who can't guess correctly which wines have more body and which less, even if no one has ever defined it for them. They just "feel it." And it's fortunate that they do, since it's among the most important qualities when it comes to determining which wines they'll enjoy in a particular situation.

The Importance of Feelings

Another of the most readily identifiable attributes of a wine is its texture, which is simply whether it feels viscous, smooth or rough. You can develop a feeling for body and texture in a wine even more easily and naturally than you can develop a feeling for balance, which itself isn't hard, as we've already seen. Yet, with an understanding of body, texture and balance, you'll have mastered all the elements that wine professionals consider most essential in evaluating a wine.

Very talented taste professionals dissect the taste of coffee, tea and other comestibles much the way a wine critic dissects wine, but consumers don't usually feel the need to emulate them. It's easy to see why others shouldn't expect to match the skills of these experts. They're carefully trained, adapt their whole lifestyle to the needs of their profession and regularly spend hours practicing their craft.

With wine, however, a surprisingly large base of passionate consumers takes an intense interest in the finer nuances of taste. I'd be surprised if they number more than three percent of the wine drinking public, but they avidly consume the tasting notes in various books, periodicals and newspapers and often develop rather extraordinary tasting abilities of their own. Even that small group, however, uses their highly developed tasting ability only to broaden, rather than narrow down, the list of wines they can enjoy. You certainly don't need to emulate them in order to master the basics of tasting wine and learn how to choose the wines that will work best for you. When you're trying to find a light switch, you don't normally start by sniffing around in the darkest corners of the room. You reach out for what you can feel near the doorway. With wine, it's also useful to start with things you can feel, like body, texture and balance, even if they're difficult to define or often overlooked because they seem obvious.

The reason people find it helpful to break down the taste of wine is that it helps them sort through the wide variety of available choices. By understanding the characteristic tastes of different wines, they can categorize them and make better use of them. To do this properly, however, it's more helpful to develop an understanding of the broader patterns in the taste of wines than it is to concentrate on a wider and wider array of discrete tastes. Indeed, the subtler nuances of taste take on significance only after you become familiar with the larger, more readily identified taste elements that aren't found in isolated details, but in the totality of the experience.

Sorting Out Your Palate

In my initial efforts to gain an understanding of wine, I relied on many different sources. I couldn't put what they were telling me in context, however, since I didn't have many coherent thoughts of my own. It was also difficult for me to sort out the disparate biases, personal and regional preferences and, at times, hidden financial interests. Sometimes, what was the same actually seemed different because of the way it was presented. I also had a relatively simplistic notion that the best wines would simply be those that had more of whatever it was that made wines good. It didn't really occur to me that what might make one wine good might make another bad.

With such a muddled notion of what was good or bad in wine, I remained a hesitant wine consumer for many years. It wasn't until I learned to sort out my own particular taste preferences that I could put the opinions of others in context. Then I began to appreciate that what I liked in a wine usually depended more on my personal preferences than on any abstract principle someone else could explain to me. It also depended more on the overall experience than any specific attribute teased out by understanding the dynamics of my taste buds. It was necessary for me to step back a bit in order to see what was important.

Once you step back and take a moment to consider it, you'll realize that there's quite a bit more to your palate than just your tongue. Your sense of taste involves not just the sensations picked up by your taste buds, but also those sensed by the olfactory epithelium, a patch of "smell buds," as it were, high up at the back of your nose. Since the process of fermentation creates alcohol and other volatile substances, wine releases aromas more actively than most of the things we eat and drink. When it's been properly made, stored and served, the scent it releases is pleasant and delicious. Sometimes, it can be ethereal.

The aroma of a wine is often as important, and sometimes more important, to the overall taste of a wine, than the sweet, salty, bitter or prickly sensations that we sense on our tongue. But we don't taste with our mouth and nose alone. Our brain perceives taste and, as the repository for our memory bank of past perceptions, plays the most important role in our taste experience. It doesn't interpret the sensory impressions from our nose and tongue in isolation, but in the context of all the information we've stored away about things we've tasted in the past. By integrating the sensations we receive at any particular time with our memories of the past, it allows us to make comparisons and sort out what's different from what's familiar.

It's the information in your brain that creates your unique palate and forms your general taste preferences. Even if you've never tasted a sip of wine, you can know something about the wines your palate will prefer. Simply think about the tastes you like in other things:

Do you have a sweet tooth or a preference for things that are sour?

Do you prefer intense, fruity tastes or earthy, vegetal tastes?

Do you enjoy or have an aversion to greasy foods?

Do you prefer your food thoroughly cooked, lightly cooked or fresh?

Do you tend to prefer your food plain or spicy?

Are you a picky eater who has always tended to prefer a narrow range of foods or do your tastes tend to change frequently?

Are you a person who has strong preferences for certain foods and drinks, or is your taste more adventuresome?

Knowing the answers to these questions will help you make better use of this book and understand your own reactions to various wines. Metabolism, physiology and medical conditions can also affect your palate. Perhaps you're a smoker, suffer from acid reflux or take medications that change the way things taste. Don't forget this when you hear or read about the way a wine is supposed to taste.

Although wines are very adaptable, you'll enjoy them most when their tastes coincide with your own, especially if your tastes are unusual. No book can tell you what wines you'll enjoy most, only someone who understands your particular taste preferences can do that. The wines you'll enjoy most are those that reprise and complement the tastes you like most and bring them out in the foods you eat. If you have a sweet tooth, don't force yourself to drink drier wines just because others prefer them. Just be happy that there are many sweeter-tasting wines for drinkers like you and that, if you suddenly develop a taste for drier wines, there will be many new wines for you to enjoy.

"New-World" vs. "Old-World" Palates

In the world of wine today, there is much talk about "old-world" versus "new-world" wine styles and the supposed palates these different styles of wine appeal to. I doubt that anyone has a palate that's strictly one type or another, nor is it easy to imagine exactly what an old-world or new-world palate might be, but to get a general sense of your personal orientation it can help to understand why people make a distinction between "old-world" and "new-world" wines and ponder the taste profiles they might be thinking of when they use those terms.

Wines from many of the world's up-and-coming wine regions taste different from those produced in the long-established wine regions of Europe because these areas are drier. The vines are less susceptible to certain troublesome pests, but growers must irrigate, which is generally prohibited in the most prominent wine-growing areas in Europe. The prohibition against irrigation serves two objectives. Since producers often purchase grapes from growers by weight, they prefer not to buy bunches that have been bulked up with water. Relying on what nature produces keeps all growers on a level playing field and eliminates the temptation to generate·kilos at the expense of flavor.

The other benefit of restricting water at ground level is that it forces the vines to put down deep roots in order to bring up water from underground aquifers. This water tends to be rich in minerals, which add stony, earthy flavors and give the wine a characteristic sometimes referred to as "backbone."

In regions where it isn't possible to bring up water from deep underground, growers have learned other ways to enhance and add complexity to the fruit flavors in wine. These fruit flavors might be tempered in more traditional wines so as not to compete with the earthy, mineral tastes people have come to look for in them. Techniques such as planting multiple clones of a particular grape variety or the use of "designer" yeasts during fermentation have allowed winemakers to create a more fruit-forward style of wine that many people enjoy. The use of riper grapes, which have more sugar and thus give the wine a higher alcoholic content, also tends to be a characteristic of a new-world style.

You can use these broad distinctions in style to help you find the wines best adapted to your own palate. Winemakers who emulate the restrained old-world style will produce drier wines with more noticeable acidity and bitter accents. (Although traditionally produced in Europe, wines of this style can be made elsewhere with the right conditions.) Wines made in a new-world style will have more sweetness and bolder fruit flavors, as has been customary for most wines produced in North and South America, Australia, South Africa and New Zealand.

Unless you've had extensive exposure to other foods, you'll probably find that the strongest instincts of your palate are those formed during your childhood and that your tastes are heavily influenced by foods that were readily available where you grew up. This isn't always just a function of where you lived in your youth. If you lived in America, but come from a first-generation European immigrant family, you're likely to find that you prefer old-world style wines. If you grew up in an Asian community in

Europe, you may prefer new-world wines, even though you grew up in the old world.

The increasing awareness throughout the world of the great cuisines of Asia and the Middle East has challenged but not eliminated the usefulness of thinking in terms of new-world vs. old-world palates. As more and more fine restaurants feature the cuisines of Asia and the Middle East (or new cuisines blending elements of East and West), their managements are searching for wines that complement those cuisines. In addition, the increasing development of a middle class in China and India has reawakened the culture of wine in these countries, with new vineyards being planted and their traditional wines being rediscovered.

The increasing global prominence of Asian and Middle Eastern cuisines is useful to keep in mind as you develop an awareness of your own preferences, but shouldn't necessarily make it necessary for you to seek out a completely new style of winemaking. Remember that the primary stimulus for new-world wine styles has been the development of new technologies and the spread of vineyards into drier areas. Ultimately, the idea of a new-world palate represents only a greater readiness to accept the kind of wine these areas produce and the foods that go with them. In my experience, most people have the ability to enjoy both.

It's also worth remembering that the Middle East was the cradle of wine as well as civilization. The Greeks and then the Romans spread the culture of wine throughout Europe, and they spread much of Middle Eastern culture with it. The elegant, delicately spiced cuisines of the Middle East were a source of inspiration for the haute cuisines of Europe, and immigrant cultures from the Middle East and Asia continue to influence the European palate and inevitably, its wines. Meanwhile, the Asian palate, with its emphasis on bold flavors, spices and contrasts between sweet and sour, lends itself well to bolder, new-world style wines.

Since we tend to share wine more often than we drink it alone, you'll ultimately need to take into account preferences other than your own. You may have more of an old-world palate while someone you're entertaining has more of a new-world palate. You may also face the daunting task of choosing a wine for many people making individual selections from a varied menu. But whether you're choosing wines for yourself or other people, it's necessary to understand your own palate first or you'll be choosing in a way that's divorced from taste. You are the only one who can thoroughly understand the tastes you experience. The degree to which you can use that understanding to increase your own enjoyment or that of others will depend on how firmly you hold it in your grasp.

The Tools of Taste

Anything as subjective as the taste of wine can't be truly understood in the abstract; it has to be experienced. Before you can make sense out of what someone else tells you about the differences between the taste of one wine and another, you'll need to have a frame of reference: a clear set of concepts in your own mind to connect to what you're hearing. With a bit of attention, that can easily be developed as you taste various wines from time to time.

The next time you have an opportunity to taste a wine without too many distractions, try to put a name, any name it suggests to you, on whatever seems most intriguing in the wine. You don't have to do this alone. Tasting wine with someone else who's willing to start with a blank slate and is good at free association can be great fun and give you twice as many chances to come up with a concept that sticks in your memory.

Whether you're sampling alone or with others, you'll want to concentrate on a taste that seems distinct to you, so you can find it again. Once you put your own label on it, you're beginning to categorize that taste. Gradually, you'll refine your concept of what the taste is, stripping away components you later learn to place in other categories. As the various distinct tastes you recognize become more numerous, they'll begin to serve as a lens through which distinct patterns emerge, and eventually those patterns will start to converge with what you've heard others say about the taste of wine.

At that point, you won't need to worry so much about being overly influenced by what you hear, since your own framework is something you never lose once you start to build it. Some of the tastes you identify will be ones others don't talk about, because your frame of reference is unique. You're also likely to identify tastes that simply aren't the most engaging things to talk about in a wine. As long as you experience them, however, you won't forget them. They'll become part of your personal relationship with wine.

When I first started to develop my own sense of taste, I found a taste in some red wines that reminded me of unripe blackberries. Of course, that's very different from the jammy, ripe blackberry taste often mentioned in tasting notes and I soon learned to separate it from the taste of blackberries. For a while, I considered that the taste might be what others referred to as "bell pepper," but I gradually began to distinguish it from the more harmonious and pleasant bell pepper taste as well. Ultimately, it turned out that what I tasted was simply unripe grapes.

It's rare that a wine writer will mention the taste of unripe grapes. If a review mentions it, it will offend the producer, but if the review doesn't mention it, the consumer will be offended. So the politic thing to do is simply not rate these wines. If you're like me, however, and like to noodle through unrated wines looking for a bargain or just something different, it's a helpful attribute to be able to pick out.

Now that you've learned to take the time to notice them, you're ready to begin picking out your own tastes in various wines and build a set of benchmarks to use for future reference. As part of this process, you'll not only need to be able to recognize tastes, but learn how to remember them. You can significantly improve your ability to do both of these things merely by taking a few simple steps before you taste a wine. These are the basic tools of the wine taster's trade and they don't take long to learn.

Looking Good and Tasting Better

Since your palate involves more than just your tongue, it's always useful to engage all the senses as you begin to taste a wine, including your sense of sight. Before you do anything else, simply take a moment to look at the wine. Its color and consistency can tell you many things. In general, the deeper and more opaque the wine is, the more pronounced the flavor. Wines also tend to have colors that can correspond to the flavors in them. A very white wine is usually austere and bone-dry. Wines that have a tinge of green sometimes have a taste of crabapple in them, while those that are more yellow may taste like lemons or pineapples. Oak imparts a browner hue to a wine that's somewhat reminiscent of the vanilla flavor it adds to the taste. A bright red wine often tastes like red berries, while a more purple hue might be a hint that plummy notes are lurking in the taste.

Nuances of color are often most noticeable in the brighter area, or meniscus, near the rim. This is easier to see if you tilt the glass and hold it against a white background. A large area of clear liquid near the edge suggests a wine that's losing its flavor. If the color is deep right up to the edge, the wine can be expected to taste fresh and youthful. A brownish meniscus can be a sign either that the wine has oxidized excessively and will taste like vinegar or that it's achieving a graceful maturity, where the flavors will be soft and delicate. Even though these are quite different tastes, being prepared for them can help you assess how they might affect the other flavor elements in the wine. In a mature wine, for example, fruit flavors will have the subtle intensity of dried fruit rather than the vibrancy of fresh fruit.

If the surface of a wine has a lustrous shine, it's an indication that the wine is higher in alcohol. A wine that's lost most of its luster is likely to have matured a bit too much. If you swirl the wine in your glass, you can see whether it has legs—drippy lines that form along the side of the glass. The thickness of the legs and the slowness with which they cascade back into the wine is an indication of glycerin content, which shows whether the wine was produced in a warm climate where the grapes can produce both a high levels of alcohol and residual sweetness.

You can also tell a few things about a wine simply by looking at the bottle. Wines made to age for more than eight to ten years are traditionally sold in bottles with pronounced "shoulders," often referred to as "Bordeaux" bottles. The shoulders are intended to catch the sediment that drops to the bottom of the wine as it ages and would otherwise float gradually out through the neck of the bottle as the wine is poured. Even though wines are being made to be drunk earlier these days, before any significant sediment has built up, you can still expect wines in these bottles to be full-bodied and chewy from higher levels of tannin.

Bottles with the more tapered shape of the classic "Burgundy" bottle generally contain wines made to be consumed before significant sediment builds up in the bottle. They tend to be light- to medium-bodied and have the more straightforward flavors we associate with fresh fruits. The tallest and thinnest bottles, on the other hand, like those used for most Rieslings, are designed to minimize contact between air and the wine remaining in the bottle as they are emptied. This preserves their delicate aromatic qualities, so be ready to stop and smell the flowers when you drink from them.

Many of the tricks that "blind" tasters use to identify wines actually involve *looking* at them carefully before tasting them. A careful look at both the bottle and the wine in the glass can give you a good sense of what to expect long before the wine touches your tongue.

Sniffing Things Out

The next step a serious taster takes before sipping a wine is to sniff it. When you do this, it's important to draw the aroma high up into the olfactory epithelium, that little area high up at the back of the nose. By drawing the scents from a wine high up in the nose, you'll experience it the same way you do when the aroma floats up from the back of your mouth just after you swallow. It helps me to take two short sniffs followed by a long one, but be careful not to overdo it or you'll overload the circuits.

The scent of a wine can confirm or complicate the impression you get by looking at it. Young wines can barrage you with fresh fruit smells, while the delicate floral scent of an older wine can reassure you that the pale brown seeping into its color is the result of proper aging, rather than spoilage. (In well-aged wines, aroma is often referred to as "bouquet" because the scents tend to be less fruity and more floral.)

Wines that are too cold give off less scent, tipping you off that they'll taste better if you give them time to warm up. In a warmer wine, the absence of aroma signals that it's likely to be light-bodied and less flavorful. For a tannic, age-worthy wine, a lack of aroma is usually a sign that it's not ready to drink, because the tannins haven't broken down enough to let its delicate aromas emerge.

Experts often divide the aromas in wine into three distinct types. The first are the fruity and flowery scents derived from the grape variety used to make the wine. The second are those that result from the way the wine is made. So, for example, wines aged in wood can have smells that remind you of cedar shavings, vanilla or toast. The final grouping is the most complex, because it involves the subtle and complex aromas derived from aging. These gradually replace more vivid fruit scents with deeper, sweeter scents, reminiscent of dried fruits, flowers and gentle spices.

Often, the scent of an unfamiliar wine will seem rather strange to you. Many people find the ammonia smell in a fresh Sauvignon Blanc, the faint whiff of petrol given off by a classic Riesling or the musty odor of well-rotted manure given off by an earthy Pinot Noir unsettling. However unusual and downright weird these aromas are, they're tip-offs to tastes many connoisseurs consider characteristic expressions of these grape varieties and can help explain why what you're drinking might carry a price many times above the competition. Being prepared to expect these tastes can help you avoid being thrown by the taste of the wine and rejecting it out of hand. If you're expecting something unusual, you can accept it more readily and see if the winemaker has been able to knit it together with the wine's other elements into a harmonious expression of the vine.

The cues you pick up by looking more carefully at the wines you're about to drink and taking a moment to absorb their aromas will prepare you to sort through what you taste and place it in a better context by making connections between what you're tasting and the impressions and memories that are, in the last analysis, your true palate. Engaging the mind in placing these tidbits of taste in a broader context also helps us connect with a more abstract, but no less important quality of wine—its ability to free us from the obvious and make us conscious of our ability to comprehend the complexities of life in a more relaxed, refined and less threatening way. Putting aside the instinct to consume it compulsively allows the wine to help us float a bit above the surging tides of life, place our day-to-day cares in a broader context and become more receptive to possibilities we might otherwise bar from our consciousness as unwelcome distractions.

Developing Your Routine

You can learn a great deal by taking the time to visually examine various wines and sample their aromas. Both steps are important and can be continued as you drink a wine, even occasionally becoming the focal point for your enjoyment of a wine during a quiet respite alone or with friends. But they are not an end in themselves, as many seem to believe. Mastering all the shades of color that different wines can have is useful if you enjoy beating other people in blind tastings, but it doesn't change the taste of the wines you enjoy, while sniffing away repeatedly can be overdone to the point that it becomes useless to you and annoying to other people. Ultimately, these steps will be most helpful if you can use them discreetly whenever you drink wine. With a little practice, you can learn to incorporate them into your routine and perform them subtly, without taking more than a brief pause from whatever else the occasion demands. Once you do, you'll notice others doing it as well. They may even give you a knowing glance.

Taking the time to look at and smell a wine before you taste it is like the set-up routine a golfer or free-throw shooter uses when addressing a shot. It allows you to put aside any distractions of the moment, experience the taste of the wine in a broader context and connect it with the memorable wines you've tasted before. Once you get the hang of it, it becomes as instinctive as blowing softly on a steaming cup of coffee and shouldn't require more than a few moments. Those moments are crucial to your ability to develop reference points so you don't taste wine in a vacuum. Consciously and subconsciously, you'll start to sort out the differences between wines. By preparing your mind for what might be coming, you'll allow yourself to observe as well as experience the taste of a wine and store your impressions away for future use.

As you begin to appreciate and employ all the physical and mental processes that influence your sense of taste, you'll be better able to discern the differences among wines and make judgments about the wines you taste. Your memories of what you've enjoyed will become more firmly established and remind you of things that could be there, but aren't: a weightier feeling on your tongue, more rounding of the harsh edges, a certain intensity of flavor. You'll begin to know why a certain wine leaves you feeling a bit unsatisfied and another delivers contentment.

You'll also find that some of the inexpensive wines on the shelf at your local grocery chain or in the remainder bins of wine shops do quite well for your everyday needs. Pay attention to those that complement your favorite meals and snacks. Here's another virtue in the diversity of wine: as you learn how modest wines can better suit your everyday needs, you can enjoy them more, while saving higher-priced wines for the special occasions they were bred for.

In the beginning, building up your mental wine database may require you to take a few moments away from just enjoying the sheer pleasure of your wine, but the time required will diminish quite quickly until it becomes almost unnoticeable. Eventually, the process of comparing new wines to the ones you've experienced in the past will become instinctive and you'll find yourself developing a good general sense of what various wines will taste like before you drink them.

Having that general sense helps the subtler nuances of a particular wine stand out and become easier to remember. You'll gradually find it easier to make your own judgments about what you and others like and, as you become more familiar with the wines you enjoy, you'll notice that they work better in some situations than others. You can use this knowledge to think strategically about the wines you choose for any particular occasion, so they can maximize the pleasure they provide to you and others. But to make the most of this, you'll need to avoid the temptation to become too enamored with your early successes.

Many wine drinkers are tempted to stick with a favorite wine once they find it. They also narrow their choices by relying too heavily on ratings or becoming unduly focused on the wines of a particular region before they understand what else is available to them. Let's examine some of these issues in more detail so that, by keeping your field of view large enough for a proper perspective, you can use your tasting skills to best advantage.

Playing Favorites

How to avoid the crowds

With all its abundant variety, its well-recognized adaptability and its ability to bring a pleasant surprise to the dreariest of days, wine can add more than a little spice to our lives. Why would anyone want to turn drinking it into a dull routine?

Once, at the apartment of a wealthy New York businessman, I appreciatively accepted a glass of a very sought-after cult wine from the Napa Valley region in California. After presenting it to me, he asked how I liked it (very much, thank you) and then mentioned with feigned offhandedness that it was the only wine he ever drank. Obviously, he was making a statement about his wealth, not his taste.

My slightly pretentious friend may have been fibbing a bit about his wine-drinking habits, but many people fall into the rut of drinking the same type of wine over and over again. Why they do it isn't really such a mystery. Although they may have tried to learn more about wine, they've found it intimidating and are trying to stay in their own comfort zone. One thing you can be sure of is that most of them don't understand as much about wine as you do after reading the last few chapters. Otherwise, they wouldn't be so intimidated.

Many years ago, I attended an introductory-level wine tasting. A wide range of wines was being presented, consisting of about six whites and six reds with diverse characteristics. Our gifted leader had a wonderful talent for making people feel comfortable asking the most basic questions about wine and engaged the audience in a lively dialogue.

About two-thirds of the way through the session, the fellow in front of me, who'd previously been silent, burst out "That's the one I like!" Although the presenter gave him an encouraging smile, I thought I could see the disappointment on her face. He'd missed her basic point: no one wine is right for every occasion or will always satisfy anything as fickle as our taste. Several minutes later, she told the group, or perhaps she intended it just for him, that she'd never met a wine she didn't like.

I could understand both the disappointment of the instructor and the instinct of the gentleman in front of me. She was looking to expand the horizons of her audience and get them to understand how much variety wine had to offer. He had lost his bearings in all that variety, however, and was looking for an anchorage.

This type of reaction reminds me of an old joke one of my uncles used to tell about an Italian artisan who had come to New York to take a job in a small workshop. Each day, the workers would break for lunch and go to a luncheonette down the road. Unfamiliar with English, he went hungry for a few days because he couldn't order. Then his co-workers taught him how to order beef stew. He proudly ordered beef stew for a few weeks until he began to tire of it, so he asked his friends to teach him how to order a ham sandwich. When he ordered the ham sandwich, however, the waitress asked him if he'd like it on white or rye. After thinking for a moment, he replied the only way he knew how—"Beef stew!"

Stuck in a Rut

We all need a wine we can turn to the way the poor soul in my uncle's joke fell back on his beef stew, a wine that handles most of our everyday needs and can serve as a bit of a refuge when we're just too worn out to go looking for adventure. If we rely on a single wine too much, however, we can fall into a rut and never get enough experience with other wines to learn the things they can do better. It's also easy to settle on a favorite wine prematurely, long before we really know what we need to have in such a trusted companion.

It's a fundamental mistake to think any single kind of wine could be best for you. Yet it's a common misconception that all wines should be measured against a single set of benchmarks to determine whether they are good or bad. When you think this way, it seems logical that there's just one wine you need to find: the best you can afford.

In fact, what's best for us is always changing, and no one wine should be expected to serve all our needs better than all others. In the early stages of learning about wine, we don't tend to appreciate this, because we experience the taste of the wines we drink only in the broadest outline. If we're introduced to a wine under favorable circumstances, we form a good first impression, but if the circumstances aren't ideal, we tend, unfairly, to blame the wine. We may be dimly aware that our preferences vary with the weather, the setting or the foods we're eating, but we don't appreciate the degree to which these can influence us. So if we don't find a wine appealing, we tend to cross it off our list, and commence a downward spiral in which the wines we value fall into a narrower and narrower range.

If we focus our efforts on the search for "better" before we develop a proper understanding of what wine really is, we may find a few that appeal to us broadly and tend to assume that there is an inherent characteristic in these wines that makes them "good." If it seems to be the grape variety, then we limit ourselves to the wines made from that variety; if it seems to be a particular region, then we stick to that region. For many people, this increasingly narrow-minded view of wine occurs so naturally as to seem right, but it will leave you with some dangerous misconceptions.

Lost in the Crowd

Another reason people drink the same wines over and over is that they rely on newspaper columns, magazines, television shows and blogs to provide them with wine information. The core audience for these media outlets is a knowledgeable group of consumers looking for something new and exotic. Like passionate followers of music and art, these adventuresome wine lovers are comfortable with their knowledge of the standard repertoire and are looking for something new and different. Keeping up with them is a bit like trying to learn about music by listening to the latest avant-garde composers.

For some reason, even less adventuresome consumers are curious about wines they can never drink. So the media has a tendency to talk about either the most legendary or most obscure wines and pays less attention to the great bulk of wines in the middle. As a result, most of the information provided by the media about wines that are readily available to the average consumer comes in the form of advertisements and commercials. This isn't really anyone's fault; the media is just focusing on what the audience is most interested in and what their sponsors are trying to promote.

The media also tends to focus on people and things that have already become household names. If you're a struggling young commentator trying to make a mark, an article about what esteemed French and American chefs say about the relative merits of legendary wines from Bordeaux and Napa Valley is more likely to get noticed than the most insightful article you could write about ordinary people drinking ordinary wine.

Few people are lucky enough to permanently inhabit the wine stratosphere, and most who do are wine writers and restaurant critics. For them, the subtle differences in the Burgundian soil in the few feet between the vineyards of La Tâche and Romaneé-Conti is a matter of endless fascination. For the rest of us, it's escapist fantasy.

There's a degree to which the *Wine Spectator, Decanter* or *Food and Wine* magazines are tabloids and the most highly recognized domain wines are celebrities. We don't read about the famous and the freakish because we need to learn to live like them; we're just susceptible to fantasy and fascinated by horror. Similarly, it can be entertaining to read about wines we can't drink; it just doesn't do much to advance our basic understanding of wine. The most sought-after qualities of great or obscure wines aren't those we need to appreciate in order to understand the vast majority of wines we can actually get our hands on.

To be fair, most wine publications do make a considerable effort to provide their readers with information about good values in less expensive wines. But they and their advertisers clearly understand our fascination with the great estates and the more outsized personalities in the world of wine, so their content reflects this. That's worthwhile to keep in mind when you read them.

It's also worth remembering that, just as ordinary people can be quite interesting once you get to know them, many less glamorous wines can have great depth of personality and be fascinating themselves. All you really need to do to get to know them is spend some time with them. Take advantage of what you've learned about the basic structure of wine and how to taste it. The more you get to know about the wines you drink regularly, the better prepared you'll be to appreciate something different.

The Classic Progression

It takes far too long, but the average consumer does build a familiarity with wine by drinking the more well-known and widely available wines and eventually will become familiar with some of the lesser-known ones. Still relatively young, the progression of the American wine market mirrors the kind of progression that wine lovers typically go through as they begin to learn about wine. Following prohibition in the 1920s, economic depression in the 1930s and wars in the 1940s, 50s and 60s, American consumers first began to seek out and be willing to pay for something out of the ordinary in wine in the 1970s. Initially, most of the attention was given to wines made with Cabernet Sauvignon and Chardonnay grapes, the grapes associated with the legendary red wines from Bordeaux and white wines from Burgundy that Thomas Jefferson recommended to Americans, which had finally begun to dominate the American market for imported wines.

After George Taber spread word in *Time* magazine that a 1976 tasting in Paris had ranked California wines on a par with legendary French wines, Americans became more comfortable making their own decisions. First a Merlot craze hit the market; then, as chronicled by the movie *Sideways*, Pinot Noir became the next big thing. Moving back to whites, the American market fixated briefly on Viognier, then the mainstream moved on to Sauvignon Blanc and Pinot Grigio. Meanwhile, the expanding market harbored growing cults worshiping Zinfandel, Shiraz, Cabernet Franc, Riesling, Grüner Veltliner and Malbec.

Today the wine media covers a vast array of different wines. Consumers around the world are flooded with information about up-and-coming wine regions and small artisanal producers whose wines are almost impossible to find. As the media struggles to keep the attention of a core audience that's searching for the next new thing, it's understandably becoming more difficult to connect with average consumers and help them learn the basics.

Although there's value in learning about different wines one at a time, what's fashionable at any given point may not be the easiest thing for starting wine drinkers to connect with, and all the buzz and hype about something you aren't ready to deal with can be distracting. When everyone is praising a certain type of wine and you find it a bit strange, you might get the impression that you don't really like wine as much as other people or feel better off just sticking with an old favorite regardless of what anyone else says. Either way, it's easy to become discouraged.

How to Chart Your Own Course

It's a bit counterintuitive, but there's a quicker and less confusing way to expand your wine horizons than following the fashions of the wine media. Just as taking time with a few glasses of wine can help speed up the process of understanding the basics, concentrating on just one or two types of wine in the beginning can speed up the process of understanding a broader and broader range of wines in the end.

The reason I've been warning you about the dangers of becoming starstruck with the latest wine celebrity or clinging too closely to an old favorite is precisely because I'm about to tell you to narrow your focus, and I don't want you to do it the wrong way. By showing you how to taste your wines better, I've set you up for a potential disaster, since it can be overwhelming to experience all the different tastes that a wide range of wines can exhibit. Faced with too many different wines, you'll have too many things to keep track of, so you'll need a way to keep them sorted out.

If you approach the process logically, however, it isn't all that difficult to become familiar with the various tastes of many different wines. You just need to start by getting thoroughly familiar with the wines made from one or two grape varieties, so you can use them as reference points. By focusing intently on these, you'll be able to avoid distractions and become thoroughly familiar with the taste of those wines. Then it will be relatively easy to expand your horizons by comparing them to other wines.

Starting your adventures in wine with one or two grape varieties will allow you to see how climate and winemaking techniques influence the taste of wine. Rather than haphazardly following the fashions of the wine media, you'll be able to concentrate on these important elements of taste and see that they are predictable. And as you learn to predict the elements of taste that climate and winemaking technique impart to a wine, you'll be preparing yourself to move on to wine made from other grape varieties, since you'll be able to separate the unique tastes these varieties contribute from the taste elements that cross over from one variety to another.

So before you focus on the latest new thing that the wine media is buzzing about, make sure you really understand the wines you already enjoy. Take two of them: perhaps a red and a white. Be sure you know where they're made and what grapes they're made from. If this information isn't available on the label or from the person you usually buy them from, it might be available online or perhaps you have a friend who might know. You could even contact the producers, since they usually enjoy hearing from people who like their wine.

When you have this information and a quiet moment to taste the wines without distractions, take a good sip of one and then the other. Remember to look at each wine, swirl it around in the glass and take a good sniff before you put it in your mouth. Take some time to think about the first wine when you finish your first sip and ask yourself why you like it. When you try the second wine, ask yourself what's different about it. Don't worry about finding two wines that are very different. People are usually surprised at how different any two wines are when they taste them side by side.

As you compare the two wines, some of the taste differences will seem rather easy to put your finger on, particularly if the wines have distinctly different fruit flavors. Others will be harder to identify and difficult to give a name to. But as you start to sort through the differences, one thing will become apparent: there are many of them. You won't be able to categorize wines by taste, unless you can organize the myriad taste elements into recognizable patterns. Learning to pick apart, one by one, all the many taste characteristics of any wine is an impossible task. But you can learn to recognize the more obvious elements of taste and organize the others into broad groups associated with particular wines.

Understanding Body and Texture

The best way to begin organizing your tasting experiences into coherent patterns is to build on what you've already learned about how balance, body and texture affect the taste of wines. While exotic flavors often take center stage in descriptions of a wine's taste, it's the body and texture of a wine that serve as the cast and crew behind these leading actors, while balance provides the performance space.

As we've seen, body and texture are the tactile impressions a wine gives us. Most of the terms used to describe them seem either unexciting or slightly malevolent, such as weight, heat, dryness, bite and grip. When a wine is described as "medium-bodied" or "crisp," these characteristics don't seem like things you need to look for as much as things that will be obvious. This is why they're easy to ignore, since we don't tend to concentrate on things that are obvious; but it's also why they're good traits to start with as you look for the characteristics that distinguish one wine from another.

Because they're easy to sense, body and texture are actually the best things to concentrate on as you begin to build your wine knowledge. They reveal a wine's "structure," which tells how the winemaker molded the raw material of grapes into a finished product. The effort to bring structure to a wine can influence the winemaker's decisions about when to harvest, how to control fermentation, where and how long to age a wine and many other decisions essential to the final taste.

The uninitiated are understandably nonplussed when some-one hands them a glass of something liquid and starts talking about structure. But when they hear that it relates to easily recognized things like "weight" or "roughness" they tend to think: "Sure, I get it. Is that all there is to it?"

The mouth-filling sensation of a full-bodied wine may be easy to recognize, but the process that creates it is very dynamic. What does most to create the impression of body is the sensation of heat, something we tend to associate more with fiery distilled spirits rather than wine because it comes from alcohol. This isn't a particularly pleasing sensation for most people, which is why they sometimes screw up their faces when they drink straight liquor.

Wines with lower alcohol levels seem lighter-bodied because they don't fill the mouth with the warm taste of alcohol the way a full-bodied wine does, but the sting of alcohol will still be noticeable unless there's something else in the mix. This is where the basic sweet and sour qualities of the wine that I first asked you to concentrate on become important. For any wine to seem pleasant, it must retain enough residual sugar and acidity to stand up to the alcohol it contains. But the alcohol in the wine is produced by fermenting away the sugar in the juice, reducing the very sweetness needed to stand up to the alcohol and serve as a counterpoint to sour taste derived from the wine's acidity. This is why balance isn't merely a question of sweet vs. sour, or fruitiness vs. acidity.

A wine becomes attractive when all the major elements of structure achieve a dynamic equilibrium and create a body that's well proportioned. In this sense, the soul of a wine is in its body, and is tri-partite, like Plato's vision of the human soul. It reveals itself in the dynamic tension between its spirited alcohol, desirable fruit and disciplined acidity.

The Durability of Structure

As a counterpoint to a wine's sweetness and a foil for the heat generated by its alcohol, acidity plays the leading role in giving a wine structure. When a wine's acidity is strong, it adds to the feeling of body, and keeps our flavor instincts alive by making the wine seem more neatly defined and focused. It helps preserve the freshness of the wine while it's stored and keeps its taste from becoming boring while we drink it. With all it can contribute to the mix, you'll find it useful to be able to gauge the amount of acidity in a wine, but that's not always as easy as judging sweetness or body. Because acidity has many different components, it can be hard to identify as a basic taste.

When I ask people to describe what they think acidity in a wine tastes like, they often use words like "crisp," "harsh" or "raw" and agree when I suggest the brisk tanginess of vinegar. Indeed, when professionals refer to an "acidified" wine, this is what they talk about as well. But this is confusing, because it isn't what they mean when they talk about acidity in wine in general. In that case, they're thinking simply of the sour taste that offsets the wine's sweetness, nothing harsh or raw at all. This sour taste comes from tartaric acid, which is by far the most dominant acid in wine.

If you taste tartaric acid in its pure form, you may not think of it as particularly acidic. Cream of tartar, which you probably already have in your kitchen, is made from the larger crystals of tartaric acid that accumulate on barrels during the winemaking process. If you have some handy, shake a bit out on your palm and lick it (it's a powder, not to be confused with tartar sauce, in which it's only an ingredient). At first it won't taste like much at all, but will leave a mildly bitter aftertaste, like the feeling you get after you've left an aspirin tablet on your tongue too long before washing it down with water.

When cream of tartar is combined with boiled sugar to make candies, they're referred to as "sours," the kind that make saliva gush out and collect under your tongue when you suck on them. In fact, the most reliable way to test a wine's acidity is to take a decent swig and notice how long it stimulates the production of saliva, the way sucking on a sour candy would. Thinking about hard candies as a kind of solid form of wine (without the alcohol, of course) can help you understand your preferences in wine better. Various hard candies have different levels of sweet and sour elements, so your preferences, now or when you were a child, can give you hints about where you fit on the sweet-sour spectrum, which is the area of taste where personal differences are most likely to be divergent. These preferences can also suggest which fruit flavors you'll prefer in wine.

You may also enjoy using cream of tartar to artificially create your own "instant wine." Add some cream of tartar to a glass of water until it has a fairly sour taste. Then add some sugar until you get a nice balance of sweet and sour. Replace the water you consumed while sampling with a few splashes of vodka, stir it, and you'll get something vaguely reminiscent of a horrible wine. If you add a little lemon or lime juice and food coloring and chill it, you might even be able to fool a few of your more gullible friends. Just don't try it with anyone who doesn't have a good sense of humor.

In wine, you're most likely to notice a dominant taste of tartaric acid in light, dry, un-oaked wines made from Chardonnay or Riesling grapes. It plays a vital role in giving all wines their basic taste. This isn't just because it's present in quantity, but also because of its unique crystalline structure. Its durable crystals make it much less susceptible than other acids to being broken down during fermentation or aging. This is why wine professionals say that, over time, the structure of a wine changes less than its flavor.

The fruit flavors associated with other acids evolve as they break down, while the sourness of tartaric acid is a more stable and ubiquitous taste in wine. Since it's always there, it's well worth learning to recognize. Once you can separate out its taste, the other more exotic and changeable fruit flavors in a wine stand out in bolder relief and become easier to identify. Soon, you'll be adding herbs, spices and other flavors well.

Rough and Tumble Tannins

Some of the many other acids in wine, particularly citric and malic acids and their by-products, do have the harsher attributes people ordinarily think of as acidic. Although these play an important role in what wine professionals refer to as the "overall acidity" of a wine, their most important contributions are to the flavor rather than the feel of a wine, so I will pass over them for now and concentrate next on tannic acid, whose main contribution to a wine is to its texture. This is so different from what other acids do that wine professionals tend to talk about tannins if they weren't acids at all. How often have you heard someone talk about the "acids and tannins" in wine as if they were two separate things? There's a reason for that.

What makes tannins so different is their interaction with the tissues in your mouth. Especially in young wines, tannins impart a textural roughness that swells the tissues and leaves the tongue and the sides of your mouth feeling scraped and dry. This helps a wine cut through fatty compounds that coat the palate and refresh it for the next bite when you eat rich foods. It adds to a wine's ability to stimulate the appetite and aid digestion, but can also interfere with our ability to discern the flavors in a wine.

Tannic acid helps to preserve wines as they age, but it's not as durable as tartaric acid, and slowly breaks down. This is useful because the complex flavors that develop in the wine over time become more accessible as its tannins break down. If an age-worthy wine is properly made, it will have a "drinking window" where its tannins will soften just in time for its fruit flavors to evolve to a point of exquisite delicacy, taking their rightful place in an overall taste experience that can only seem too fleeting. Wait too long, however, and the tannins will break down to the point where they no longer protect and articulate the wine. From that point on, the window will begin to close and the wine will become increasingly flat and tasteless.

Like the sweetness of sugar and the sourness of tartaric acid, the rough texture of tannic acid isn't hard to spot once you know what it is, and its intensity varies from wine to wine. It may not be as fashionable as picking out the exotic fruit flavors in the latest trendy varietal, but by taking the time to become familiar with these elements of structure you'll learn to spot the most important differences between various wines quickly and reliably.

While grape varieties contribute many of the varied flavors in wine, it's the interaction between those flavors and the structural characteristics of a wine that give us the stunning and subtle tastes that make some wines so exciting. These change as winemakers adjust the structure in response to local climatic conditions. Now that you understand structure, you're ready to learn how these conditions create predictable patterns in the way different wines taste. With this knowledge, you'll have a good idea what any wine will taste like before you select it, even if you've never tasted it before. Then you won't have to stick with an old favorite or use other shortcuts in a desperate and unproductive attempt to prevent a nasty surprise.

Climatic Characteristics

The grape varieties that produce wine are like Goldilocks. They don't like it too hot or too cold. So it's not surprising to find them sensitive to the subtle influences of various microclimates. Some varieties are better suited to cooler climates and others can take a bit of heat, so growers look to plant the varieties whose qualities are best suited the overall climate in the location where they'll be grown. Then the winemaker's skill can bring out the best of these qualities as they're affected by the day-to-day weather conditions and other factors that impact the wines each year.

When a cool climate is the result of latitude (i.e., more northerly or southerly, depending on the hemisphere), grapes have a shorter growing season. They will tend to have more acidity, since the ripening process has less time to break down the acids in the grapes and produce sugar. Malic and citric acids, which tend to break down more quickly than the other acids in grapes, will have a greater presence in the juice. This results in white wines that have delicate flavors like green apple and pear and red wines with flavors like raspberry, cherry and cranberry. Since these wines are lower in sugar they'll also have less glycerol content and tend to be lighter-bodied.

In a good year or a favored site, grapes in these cool-climate areas can have higher levels of sugar and more-pronounced flavors and aromas, but the flavors in the wines they make will still be lighter ones like anise, pear, and white melons, in keeping with the underlying taste complexion of the grape varieties that are best suited to cooler areas. The lower levels of sugar in grapes grown in cool-weather climates will also result in wines that are lower in alcohol. In a troublesome year, it's not uncommon for the alcohol level to be enhanced (and the acidity offset by a bit of sweetness) through the addition of grape concentrate or sugar during the fermentation process, but the overall objective will be to emulate the wines produced in the better years.

As consumers of white lightning, aguardiente, poitín, and other highly distilled spirits can appreciate, alcohol itself has a sweet taste. Since the lower level of alcohol produces less evident heat, there can be a noticeably sweet taste in lighter-bodied wines, even though little residual sugar remains after the grapes have been fermented. This accounts for the confusion many people feel when they hear Rieslings described as "dry" wines and why it's a mistake to avoid them for fear that they contain more calories than other wines. Only the late-harvest Rieslings, such as the Spätlese and Auslese versions actually contain significant amounts of residual sugar.

Where cool maritime or mountain breezes influence the climate, the firmness and acidity of the grapes can be maintained in latitudes closer to the equator. Similarly, in cooler areas, rivers and lakes can elevate temperatures and luminosity (the general brightness of an area), resulting in longer and more productive growing seasons. These allow the grapes to develop flavors like lemons, limes, grapefruit or melons in white wines and strawberries and black cherries in reds. It also produces higher levels of alcohol and residual sugar, which results in wines that are more medium-bodied.

The interplay between sweetness and spiciness becomes more of a factor as you move into warmer wine-growing areas, as the grapes can be expected to have more sugar content when harvested. Citric and malic acids, which can give wine a noticeable edge, break down quickly in hot conditions. So tartaric acid, with its more stable crystalline structure, plays a more important role in the taste of the wine, providing durable sour notes to play against the sweetness of the sugar.

Because of the higher sugar content in the grapes, dry wines made in warmer regions will contain more alcohol. To mute its prickle, the grape varieties planted in these areas will have fruit flavors that are denser and more mouth-filling. White wines will have more tropical fruit flavors, like pineapple, plum and kiwis, while red wines will exhibit wild, black fruit flavors, like blackberries, black currants (cassis) and prunes. These fruits hold up well when they are stewed or made into jam and, in a warm year, it sometimes tastes as though these fruits were stewed on the vine. These varieties also tend to produce a bit of iodine, which can give the wines a salty or "leathery" taste.

As you can see, despite significant differences between grape varieties and the styles of wines made from them, there is a discernable pattern to the tastes produced by climate. Cooler-weather wines tend to have more delicate flavors, less alcohol and a lighter feel, and their acidity is more evident even if their pH level may be higher. The whites are likely to have citrus-type flavors, while the reds tend to have "red fruit" flavors. Warmer regions produce white wines with lush, tropical flavors, while the reds have "black fruit" flavors. Both the whites and the reds from warmer areas will be heavier-bodied and, with higher levels of iodine and tannin, have saltier and drier textures. In all wines, as the alcohol content rises, the wines tend to taste and smell spicier.

Once you develop a sense of these patterns, it's easier to sort out the characteristics produced by climate and identify the unique flavors that a grape variety contributes to the wine. Whenever you taste a wine, think a bit about the climatic effects and stylistic decisions inherent in what you experience. It will eventually become instinctive for you to associate textural elements, such as body and bite, with different fruits, spices and other tastes, but it requires a bit of conscious practice to develop this instinct. For this, a certain amount of formal and informal comparison tasting helps.

Comparative Tasting

Many budding wine enthusiasts compare wines the way adolescents compare potential romantic partners. Because of their limited experience, they endow them with imaginary qualities, rate them on a crude linear scale and pretend to be familiar with ones they've never known. You can avoid going through this painful period by simply taking some of the wines you already know and using them to develop realistic relationships with other wines through comparative tastings. The wines you know best are in the best position to help you see the strengths and weaknesses of others in a one-to-one comparison.

Now that you understand the structural variations among wines based on climatic differences, you should be able to learn to spot and become more familiar with these differences among various wines when you taste them. Comparative tastings serve as a step-by-step method of assimilating your experiences in a logical way. When you find something that's intriguingly different, comparing it to an old favorite that you're thoroughly familiar with can help you figure out just what the differences are. This will make it easier for you to recall the differences later and build a framework for keeping track of them.

You can learn to distinguish geographic characteristics by organizing your tastings "horizontally"—tasting wines from different regions that were produced in the same year. Similarly, by organizing your tastings "vertically" (comparing samples of the same wine or style of wine from different years), you can learn to recognize more quickly what aging brings to a wine. You can also make comparisons between different producers, which will allow you to see the different qualities that a winemaker can create in a wine.

You needn't be in a hurry to organize carefully structured tastings. The opportunity to make comparisons should come up in the course of your normal consumption. You may notice an interesting comparison on a retailer's shelf, offered by the glass at your favorite restaurant or bar or among the wines served at a dinner party.

Stay alert and almost every occasion where there is more than one wine will be the occasion for a comparison. You'll be saying to yourself: "These two wines are from the same varietal, but different regions" or "These are from the same varietal and region, yet were made in different years." These on-the-fly comparisons are bit trickier than carefully structured verticals or horizontals, but they will still give you a chance to expand your wine knowledge. Instead of just choosing the wine you think you'll like best and sticking with it, you can try something else, make a comparison, and give yourself a chance to learn more and find something you might like better.

The comparisons you make on the fly will also be more realistic in terms of the way choices among wines are ordinarily presented to you. You don't often get the chance to try several different vintages (years of production) of the exact same wine, or even wines produced in the same vintage from different regions, nor do you need to control things quite so rigidly in order to benefit from comparative tasting. The most rigidly controlled tastings are used to tease out the subtle rather than the broad differences between wines. You can learn to spot the broad differences, and make the most rapid progress toward proficiency, by comparing almost anything.

If you're the kind of person who finds it useful to take notes, you can jot down what you've tasted as you sample various wines. You may find it useful to take a photo of the labels (or even just save your favorite empty bottles) in order to help refresh your recollections later. This can help train you to think about the taste of the wines and speed up your learning curve, but it's not a necessity. Be careful not to take notes as a substitute for thinking about the wines deeply enough to remember what impressed you most about them.

Most of us don't drink wines under circumstances where it's convenient to either take or refer to notes, so you may find it helpful to develop other ways to remember your impressions. For me, talking about what I've tasted with someone else, either at the time I taste it or at some point during the next few days, helps me remember what I've tasted better than taking notes does. My notes tend to get lost in my pockets and be illegible when they come back from the wash.

However you remember the taste of your wines, the important thing is to be able to identify the things you like and dislike and be able to associate them with wines that are readily available for you drink. It's also important to build your wine knowledge by adding to it in small increments that expand on what you already know. Wine buffs will understandably be looking for flavors that are new and surprising, but as you build your fundamental knowledge be careful not to ignore a wine's structure and the textural elements that might seem obvious.

Inner Awareness

Don't be discouraged if, in the beginning, the only wines you can compare are the wines right in front of you. The process of comparative tasting will train you to make connections between textures and flavors and develop an inner awareness of the range of tastes in different wines. This will raise your consciousness about all the wines you drink and help you remember the special ones. Soon you'll be able to compare any wine you taste to some of the memorable wines you've tasted in the past and eventually you'll begin to sort out and organize these tastes in the way that's most meaningful to you. Once you can notice the differences between what you taste and what others say they taste, you'll be able to observe, rather than follow, the fashions of the wine world. You can give the famous and the freaks the respect they deserve and not have to wonder if they're for you.

Even though the media lavishes attention on legendary and exotic wines, there's still plenty of information available to help you find the ordinary wines that are best suited to your palate. Unfortunately, much of it is in a kind of impenetrable code only knowledgeable wine drinkers understand. Later on, I'll help you learn to understand that code and show you the most important things to focus on when you read or hear something about wine. But many people look for a key to the secret code in the numbers. Before I tell you how to crack it, I have to tell you why it's not hidden in the numbers.

Playing the Numbers

Escape from the average

Some things just can't be reduced to numbers and wine is one of them. It's been said that even Isaac Newton knew better than to drink and derive, but if he had a calculus for his wine, we can be sure it was an inner one, shaped by his own experiences and the people he shared his wine with.

When you use someone else's number as the main reason to choose a wine, your expectations confine and regiment it. The wine joins a line of silent souls that can only conform or be further punished. Release it and let it run. It won't hurt you.

The instinct to buy wines by number is understandable. When dining out for a special occasion, you may want to step your wine purchases up a notch or two, but worry that you're wandering a bit out of your league. In a wine shop, the wide range of selections available can be daunting. On these occasions, a numerical ranking may seem a useful, easy-to-comprehend guideline.

Most good restaurateurs and retailers make an effort to offer helpful assistance. But many wine snobs won't deign to ask for their advice and other consumers may be too timid or suspicious to ask for it. Since they know that customers often feel in need of advice they won't ask for, they'll often display ratings given by well-recognized wine reviewers. They know it's hard to win the consumer's trust for their own recommendations because of a lurking feeling that there may be some self-interest behind the recommendation. It also may be difficult to personally taste and write up all the wines and mind the store at the same time. Better to quote a positive snippet from a well-known critic and put up the numeric score.

Getting Nothing From 100

Some critics limit their rating scale to twenty points or use a scoring system like the five-star system adopted by Michael Broadbent and Clive Coates. But the ratings most used by retailers today are based on a scale of 100 points, copying a system first devised by Robert Parker, which was instinctively recognizable to

American consumers because it reminded them of the grades that they received in school. Think about it. If your history essay can get a 98, why can't a wine?

An 18 on a 20-point scale is probably as good as a 90 on a 100-point scale, but it suffers by comparison. So retailers have learned to follow the critics who score on the 100-point scale and tend to stock the wines they score most highly. The prices of these wines follow the minute gradations in ratings to a remarkable degree.

A wine that scores 90 gets a noticeably higher price than a wine that scores 89. This implies that there's a tangible difference between the 89 and the 90. But as any knowledgeable retailer, and even the critics who assign the ratings will tell you, no one but the critic can recognize the difference between similar wines rated a few points away from each other.

It's obvious that the rating itself should not be the driving force behind your choice of a wine. Why should a critic bother to do a write-up if all you need is the rating?

Why Ratings Mean So Little

A numerical rating implies that there is a single standard for all wines at all times. In fact, what people look for in one type of wine is different from what people look for in another, so there is no one algorithm that can be used to rate all wines on a consistent basis. Moreover, a perfectly fine example of a certain type of wine might not be what will work best for you at a given point in time. You might just not like that type of wine. Or it could be the wrong choice for the occasion you have in mind. Would you serve the same wine at a funeral reception in February that you would serve for a wedding in May?

Another issue is food pairing. In most cases, you don't buy a wine to drink by itself, but for an occasion at which food is going to be served. Some wines pair well with one food and not with another. How can a single numeric score tell you how a wine will pair with the food you have in mind for a specific occasion?

A numerical score can be a judgment on a wine only at a particular point in time. While many critics have a phenomenal gift for assessing a wine's future, the progress of a wine over time still involves a number of hard-to-predict factors. Differences in shipping and storage can have a major effect on the taste of a wine. So does your decision about when to drink it. Sometimes there's just "bottle variation": significant differences between bottles of wine from the same producer and vintage, even when they've been shipped and stored the same way and are being consumed at the same time. What does all that imply about assigning a rating to a wine years before it's drunk?

When Robert Parker originally devised his 100-point system, he said he would give 50 points to every wine for just showing up. In other words, he could have used a 50-point system and a one-point difference would have been equal to a two-point difference on the 100-point scale. One wonders whether he would have felt it necessary to award half-points. Would a 97 be a 45.5?

In his original system, Parker allowed five points for color and appearance, fifteen for aroma and bouquet, twenty points for flavor and finish and ten for "overall quality." In other words, the difference between a 98-point wine and a 94-point wine could conceivably be attributable solely to his color preferences. Likewise, the entire difference between a 98-point wine and an 88-point wine could be in the ten-point fudge factor for quality. Amazingly, in the entire 100 points, only twenty were allocated to flavor and finish. Think about that for a few moments.

Putting the Numbers in Context

To be fair, Parker doesn't rate wines this way now, nor did he use his system the way I've just described for long. Today, I suspect he simply tastes a wine and compares it subjectively with all the many other wines in his prodigious mental database of similar wines. He then assigns a score based on where he thinks the wine fits in the overall hierarchy.

Since he has a well-trained palate and a prodigious memory for wines, I'm sure it's useful for him to mark down a score to use when he double-checks his impressions for consistency. There's no reason why he shouldn't share it with us, but there are many reasons why we shouldn't pay too much attention to it, especially when he himself will be the first to admit that he often changes his mind. Sometimes he revises his scores significantly as a wine matures. Moreover, it's patently obvious that his palate does not speak for every palate in the world. Even if you find him more reliable than other reviewers in recommending what you like, you won't *always* like the same things he does.

It's the consumer more than the critic who should be blamed for an over-reliance on small gradations between high scores.

Sophisticated consumers may pay some attention to critics' scores, but they won't place undue reliance on them. They get to know the preferences of the critics and have a sense of which are closest to their own. They also learn which types of wine a critic rates in a way that seems accurate to them and which types the critic rates in a more idiosyncratic way. Frequently, they will look for wines they like that haven't scored well with an influential critic in a given year, sensing the opportunity for a bargain.

When looking at wine reviews, it's far more important to find reviews that make sense to you and give you insights into the wines you drink than it is to simply look for highly rated wines. This is particularly true if you don't know whether the reviewer's ratings reflect the preferences of your own palate. If you're trying to educate your palate by forcing it to like wines that are highly rated, you're going about things backward.

Robert Parker has an extraordinary ability to communicate what he tastes by writing clear, consistent and eminently readable reviews. But if you don't read these reviews, you won't be able to tell whether you and he see the same things in a wine. It's a mystery to wine professionals how so many people can be so heavily influenced by Parker's ratings, when they've never taken the time to read his reviews.

Grade Inflation

The excessive fixation of consumers on numerical scores has caused noticeable grade inflation over the last thirty years. The leading reviewers have seen the serious economic consequences a slight drop in score can have on a producer and understandably prefer to err on the high side. Then, since the higher scores are the ones that get the most attention, up-and-coming reviewers feel pressure to rate wines as highly as what they consider comparable wines rated by others.

Savvy consumers can take advantage of this. The difference between a 90 and a 94 doesn't necessarily justify a 20 percent increase in price. Moreover, the closer you get to 100 the more the score will reflect idiosyncrasies of the reviewer. Wines with these scores are not likely to be worth the price unless you share those idiosyncrasies or just like to collect highly rated wines. As you pay more attention to what you drink, you're likely to find many lower-rated or unrated wines enjoyable. Share them and you may find others getting excited about them for the same reasons you do. Isn't that more fun than sharing an expensive wine and hoping they'll enjoy it because it's on someone else's top 100 list?

Testing the Limits

You can easily judge the value of ratings for yourself now that you know how to set up comparison tastings. Simply find a few wines that are rated a few points from each other and make a note somewhere of what the ratings are. Later, when you've forgotten the ratings, pull out the wines and taste them side by side. Then go back and look at the ratings. The preferences you sensed when you tasted the wines aren't likely to reflect the gradations in ratings. You may have remarkably different reactions to these similarly rated wines or preferred a wine with a lower rating than the others. Don't assume that's because you don't know what you're doing. The rater may know much more about wine than you do, but only you know your palate.

You can also do a comparison tasting of wines whose ratings are further apart. Take one that is rated 85 and compare it to wines rated 90 and 95. Here it's more likely that your preferences will broadly coincide with the ratings, but this isn't guaranteed, especially if there is significant variation between the varietals, regions or vintages of the wines you taste.

What this last exercise suggests is that we would all be just as well off with a rating system like the one that the Michelin Guide uses for restaurants. There the vast bulk of establishments are simply deemed not worth rating, because their survival doesn't depend on superior food and service, so people won't be looking to find them in a guidebook dedicated to fine dining. Some unrated restaurants are mentioned as being worth investigating, presumably those deemed well enough above average to merit keeping an eye on. The rated restaurants are given one to three stars. These would be roughly equivalent to the 85–90, 90–95 and 95–100 ranges in the 100-point wine-rating systems. Without the one-point gradations within each of these groupings, you'd be more likely to read the review before making a choice, wouldn't you?

Whenever you see a rating, appreciate that your ability to make fine distinctions will be different from that of the reviewer. Also bear in mind that, as you shift from varietal to varietal, region to region or from one wine style to another, the degree to which your preferences will align with the reviewer is likely to change. Because change is integral to the process, the best wine for you in any given circumstance can't be predicted by a simple arithmetic scale. It will be determined by any number of interdependent factors, many of which will be personal to you or issues of the moment. To make the best choices, you'll need to develop an inner calculus that begins with who you are and what you need at a given point in time. An arithmetic scale can't begin to do the job properly.

Buying by Price

People often use a different set of numbers as a crutch in restaurants. Here the number they focus on isn't the rating, which may not be shown on the wine list, but the prices on the wine list. There usually are relationships between the prices of the wines on most restaurants' wine lists that you can use to improve your selections. They're not straightforward, however, and they bear little relationship to how much you'll enjoy the wine.

Since restaurants have an interest in whether their customers enjoy their food, they often make an effort to put wines on their list that pair well with their most popular dishes. At the same time, they have to take into account certain patterns in the way customers behave. Understanding the interplay between these factors can improve your chances of making a good choice even when you're unfamiliar with the wines on the list.

Most restaurants employ quite different strategies when they set the prices of the least expensive and most expensive wines on their list. This allows them to take advantage of the different proclivities of certain customers. They know that some customers will be more sensitive to price than they are to quality, so they pay more attention to cost than quality in their lowest-priced wines. But, if the price to the customer is low, the cost to the establishment must be that much lower in order to achieve a profit consistent with what they earn on other wines. If the customers who order these wines don't care about quality, why should the management? The issue is simply "How low can you go?"

For the highest-priced wines on the list, preserving profit margin isn't much of an issue. Some customers will want to purchase a special bottle of wine to impress someone or celebrate a special occasion. In that case, value pricing isn't likely to matter much to the target customer, who may actually feel better paying more for the wine. But a well-known name will help make the customer comfortable that the high price is justified.

Having some well-known wines on the list can also add to its luster and make the other wines on the list seem more affordable. Value pricing for these expensive wines would only increase the demand (and the cost of inventory) without doing much to improve the restaurant's profits. So it will keep only a few of these wines in stock and price them so that only people who don't care about price will buy them. These wines are there for status. They almost don't want to sell them.

The net result of the differences between splurging and budget-conscious customers is that the lowest-priced wines on the lists in many restaurants will be of questionable quality, while the more expensive wines on the list will be overpriced. In either case, the factors that dominate the pricing have little relationship to what a discerning customer should be interested in.

Sorting Through the Middle of the List

In the middle range of most restaurant wine lists, prices will be significantly higher than, but rise and fall in relation to, the cost of the wines in the general retail market. These differences in price should have little to do with which wines you should choose, however, since you should be looking for the wines that best complement the dishes you and your companions are planning to order. In the best restaurants, all the wines on the list have been chosen with this in mind, and price is obviously not the way to figure out which wines go with which dishes. Should you order a more expensive wine just because you order a more expensive dish?

If you sense that you're in a restaurant where the wines have been chosen to match certain dishes, you should be able figure out which they are. Later, I'll give you much more information about food and wine matching, but for now matching the regions of the wines on the list with the regions associated with the dishes will often narrow the choices down sufficiently. Bœuf Bourguignon obviously calls for a red Burgundy; Polpette alla Fiorentina suggests a Chianti.

Today, even restaurants without a sommelier or other staff member who specializes in wine are making an effort to hire and train staff so that they can help patrons select wines to complement the dishes they serve. A good way to tell if the restaurant does this is to ask your server if he or she is familiar with any of the wines on the list. If the management encourages them to be familiar with the taste of the wines, you're in good hands. Ask what wines they serve the staff with the dishes you're considering ordering.

Be aware, however, that only restaurants whose patrons make it worthwhile for them to care about their wines are likely to take the trouble to develop a wine list to match their menu. Many establishments serve great food, but have little call for wine. They may do a volume business for the working crowd at lunch, cater to young families with children or just be the kind of place where the average diner prefers a beer or a mixed drink. For some reason, many of these establishments feel the need to have a wine list, even though no one in the place knows much about it.

Occasionally, you may find yourself in a place that doesn't seem to have a wine-drinking crowd, but still has a fairly extensive wine list, including some wines you might recognize as having a good reputation. This isn't necessarily a sign that the wines are worth a try. Keep in mind that the more wines a restaurant keeps in stock for a beer-drinking crowd, the longer the wines will be sitting around waiting to be ordered. Unless they have a cellar, or a set of temperature-controlled wine storage cabinets, even good wines are quite likely to become seriously degraded before they're served. Be alert then, when you see half-empty bottles of wine lined up next to the liquors behind the bar, especially if they aren't being poured that much.

If you find yourself in this kind of situation, ask yourself (or better yet your waiter) where the wine cellar is. If the answer isn't convincing, don't expect too much from the wine list. Many good wines are fragile and proper shipping and storage is essential to keep them in top condition. If the person you're buying wine from doesn't seem to know that, you could end up paying good money for a wine that's gone bad, and that person isn't likely to appreciate why you're asking to send it back.

Ordering Wines by the Glass

Most restaurateurs know that budget-conscious consumers are concerned about the significant increase in the cost of a meal that may occur when a bottle of wine is included. They may recognize this when they offer wines by the glass, yet still wish to preserve their profit. They can do this by offering only less expensive wines to serve by the glass and building a good margin into the price of each glass. If they've done a good job selecting the wine, they'll be doubly rewarded when you order a second glass.

Most customers expect a wine to cost more by the glass than it does by the bottle. They appreciate the risk to the establishment of ending up with most of an unused bottle at the end of the evening. As a result, they don't expect the wines offered by the glass to be of the highest quality, just good enough not to ruin their meal. Since they can usually order the same wine by the bottle for a price lower than the equivalent number of glasses, it's fairly obvious that the higher price by the glass is not reflecting better quality, just convenience for some customers.

If you frequent an establishment where the wines by the glass are consistently well chosen, you may find it useful to order these wines by the bottle. The price is often modest in relation to what other wines on the list are offered for and a significant savings over what the same wine would cost if an equivalent quantity were ordered by the glass. You've found a place where they know how to find good inexpensive wines. Why shouldn't you both take advantage of it?

Are Expensive Wines Really Worth the Price?

Since we've seen that the price of wine can be influenced by a number of extraneous factors, you may be asking yourself whether the most sought-after wines are worth the exorbitant prices that they command in the market. It's a question I'm often asked, and my answer is that they are, but only if you can afford it.

There's plenty of very good wine that sells at ordinary prices. The differences between these wines and the most sought-after "collectibles" aren't necessarily proportional to the differences in price. Still, it's useful to understand the reasons why prestigious wines carry such high price tags. Two factors, longevity and reliability, play a legitimate role in justifying higher prices. Let's look at how they work, interact with each other, and create a spiral of escalating prices.

Longevity has long been a valuable quality in a wine. In the days before superhighways and climatization, it was difficult for a wine to stand up to the rigors of transportation and time. Being a durable wine added to its value because it expanded the market beyond the locale where the vineyard was located. Consumers also found these longer-lasting wines improving with age, since it takes time for the best characteristics of a wine to emerge. But to survive the bad influences it may be exposed to in its adolescence, a wine must be given a strong character in its youth. Making a wine that survives the rigors of time and emerges resplendent requires special handling that adds expense from vineyard to cellar.

A Place in the Sun

In any wine-growing region, the best sites are those that benefit from an ideal combination of several factors: exposure to the sun, which stimulates the production of sugar; cooling breezes, which preserve certain acids; and soil and water profiles that complement the grape varieties being grown. Since these premier sites command higher prices in the market, the wines they produce contain an inherently higher capital cost component from the point of inception.

But the cost spiral is just beginning. A grape that has desirable levels of alcohol and acidity in the vineyard is of little use to the winemaker unless it can get to the winery in that ideal state. Depending on the local weather, the window for harvesting the grapes may be anywhere from a few days to a few weeks.

Producers who pay more are in a better position to secure the massive infusion of trained labor necessary to harvest at the point of ideal ripeness. Indeed, contractors who provide vineyard labor often establish a hierarchy among their clients, offering discounts to vineyard owners who agree to pick earlier or later and charging a premium to those who insist that they come precisely when summoned.

While the cost of producing the best grapes can be considerable, there are still many tasks that must be taken care of before a bottle is coaxed gently from its slumber at the end of the long voyage from vineyard to table. Each of these provides a further opportunity to lavish time and money on the wine. Some can require a substantial capital investment.

Not all growers are in a position to own their own winemaking facilities, since a good facility can cost as much as a small vineyard. The producers who own their own facilities can whisk their grapes into the winemaking process at their peak. Others, forced to share with others or rent space from their more prestigious colleagues during downtime, don't enjoy that privilege.

In the winemaking process, tannic acids and resins add an extra measure of complexity and longevity to the wine. These can be enhanced by slower fermentation, but this is a risky process, particularly when the juice is left in contact with the skin and the stems for any extended period, because the exterior surfaces of the grape cluster are more likely to carry bacteria into the wine.

Fermentation produces the alcohol necessary to kill off harmful bacteria, but it requires a certain amount of heat to get started, and higher temperatures are more likely to help the bacteria grow. So the ability to enhance the flavor and acidity of a wine by leaving it in contact with skins and stems requires either a natural location with ideal temperature conditions or a battery of expensive temperature control equipment operated by highly skilled technicians. Now you know why wineries are sometimes referred to as "caves," even when they aren't.

The Knottiest Question

Then there is the question of the wood. Although wood is not as much of a factor in the taste of wine as it is in the taste of whiskey and other distilled spirits, it can play a significant role. In addition to providing tannins, wood contributes vanillin (from the breakdown of lignins) and caramels (from the breakdown of cellulose), which can add flavor, sweetness and mouth-feel to a wine. Most of the world's leading producers have concluded (or have been persuaded by market demand) that new oak casks are the ideal medium for storing a wine in the first crucial months after fermentation is complete. Some have even gone to great lengths to find the perfect kind of oak to match the character of their wines. But oak is a slow growing tree and the kind of oak in highest demand does not grow everywhere. As a result, the best oak casks are very expensive.

By definition a cask can only be used once before it's no longer new. Like an automobile, its value drops dramatically after first use, so the more quickly it can be pressed back into service, the more quickly its cost can be depreciated. If a winery stores its wine in a new oak cask for 8 to 10 months, it can bottle up the wine in time to put the casks to use during the next vintage, but there is no particular reason why 8 to 10 months is the ideal time for a wine to be kept in cask. A producer committed to making the best possible wine may often decide that a period from 12 to 18 months (or longer) is ideal to produce the best wine. That decision inevitably impacts the cost of one of the most expensive components in the winemaking process.

From Cask to Table

There are many other ways in which strict adherence to quality control in the vineyard and the winery can add cost to the finished product. But the price of the wine when it leaves the winery is typically less than one-third of the price a retailer will charge and one-sixth of the price it can command on a restaurant wine list. What accounts for the difference?

Not surprisingly, since it follows the pattern common for most other goods, marketing is a major component in the cost of a bottle of wine. Even though the world's leading wines are highly sought after, the process of getting the wines to the buyers who will pay the most for it involves considerable effort. Take, for a rather extreme illustration, the well-known First Growth, Château Lafite-Rothschild, which has a global reputation for quality. Only a bit more than 200,000 bottles of this coveted and collectible wine are produced each year, while *Forbes* magazine estimates that there are over 900 billionaires in the world. These lucky folks could easily afford to drink a bottle of this wine every day even though it routinely sells for more than twenty times the price of an average wine. If they did, of course, there wouldn't be enough to go around.

A number of the top producers in each of the world's wine regions compete aggressively to be king of the mountain each year. Each will dedicate a considerable portion of its revenue to brand polishing in order to maintain its lustrous image in the minds of wealthy wine drinkers around the globe. But as you might imagine, keeping the attention of a billionaire isn't easy. These producers all recognize that the value of a top brand can fade quickly if it isn't carefully nurtured. So getting top dollar for a wine actually increases its cost. Together with the high cost of quality control, this all adds up to an extremely high cost of production. From the perspective of the producer, however, the high price is defensible.

The Differential is Relative

The differential in price between the most collectible wines and others of high quality is mainly due to the relationship between their fame and their scarcity. Since higher ratings attract attention and make them better known, this relationship applies, to a greater or lesser extent, to all wines that achieve high ratings. That's why it's worthwhile to pay more attention to a wine's ability to meet your particular needs than to its price or numerical rating. After all, whatever you spend for something unsuitable is a complete waste of money, no matter how expensive it is.

Now that you've learned to take your time and use your wine-drinking experiences to become familiar with the different characteristics of the various wines available to you, you'll gradually learn how to sort through them and use them to their best advantage. Then you'll be able to choose your wines successfully without using prices or ratings as a crutch, and you'll often find, at a fraction of the price, wines you'll value as much or more than the most expensive wines. Eventually, if it hasn't already happened, you'll find yourself curled up in a quiet corner with a bottle of wine, being drawn deeper and deeper into its mysteries with every sip. The last grainy drop will leave you as unsatisfied as a lover's parting kiss. When this happens, you'll understand how impossible it is to encapsulate the experience in a number, even if it has three digits.

Investing in Real Estate

So many châteaux with so little wine!

Geography has an enormous influence on wine. It's always a good sign when the person selling you a wine knows exactly where it's from, which is usually more important than a critic's score. But location isn't the *only* thing to consider in choosing a wine. In fact, it isn't even the most important thing to consider, although you can easily get a different impression.

Some people seem to know more about the property that a wine is from than they do about the wine. For them, choosing a wine is like buying real estate: it's all about location, location and location. There are good reasons why location is important, but if you buy wines by location alone, the results can be disastrous.

Even if you've had only the briefest exposure to the traditional lore of wine, you may be aware that I'm treading on hallowed ground here. Doesn't almost every introduction to wine begin with a description of the world's principal wine-growing regions? And don't the guidebooks for every wine region provide detailed analyses of the subtle differences in the soil and microclimate among all the different wine-growing locations in the region?

You don't have to read too much about wine to get the impression that all really serious wine devotees pay at least daily homage to the importance of *terroir*: the peculiarities of soil and climate in the locations that produce the best wine. Just remember that these devotees *already* know about the taste of the grapes that go into the wines. They understand the effects of good and bad vintages, the influence that the winemaker can have on different wines and the serious flaws that can show up when wine is treated badly. Their interest in location relates to understanding specific bottles, not wine in general.

There are a number of reasons why location gets so much attention when it comes to wine. One is historical. Many of the traditions in today's wine culture come from Europe and were passed down from the Greeks and Romans. The Romans were the first to set up a bureaucratic system for classifying wines according to location. From the Greeks, they inherited not only a love of wine, but also a system of philosophy and laws based on the notion of *arête*—the inherent place of each living thing in nature. It was as obvious to them that a great wine was an expression of place as it is to us that building a successful brand requires thoughtful marketing. Since the Roman legal system classified a wine according to the place it came from, the place *was* essentially the brand and many of these brands have been consciously nurtured throughout the centuries.

Places of Grace

The importance of topography is another reason wine lovers pay so much attention to location. The best locations for growing wines tend to be on those hillsides whose slopes are angled toward the sun's zenith and have an exposure that's oriented toward the equator, but sufficiently east-facing to allow the grapes to pick up the earliest rays of the sun. Like humans, grapes prefer to take their warmth from the sun while sitting in a cool, gentle breeze and the rays of the sun make their skins darker—smoother initially, but ultimately leathery. The up-and-down movement of the air on the hillside cools the grapes in the late afternoon and naturally preserves the acidity in them as they ripen and produce sugar.

Since they tend to be rounded, however, and surrounded by other hills that can block the morning sun, hillsides rarely present broad, contiguous slopes perfectly oriented for exposure to the sun and the prevailing winds. So the most ideal locations are highly sought after and are squabbled over by heirs, or snapped up by wealthy buyers, when the opportunity arises. It's said that "A farmer covets his neighbor's land." Vineyard owners are no exception.

In any wine region, the growers, winemakers and others involved in the trade are all well aware of which locations are best. If they are lucky enough to own a choice vineyard, the extra income they can get for their grapes can allow them to afford to build a winery, an investment that most growers find hard to afford. For this and other reasons, there is a tendency for the most prestigious wines to be "domain" wines, named after a particular plot of land where the grapes are grown.

With all the attention that the top domains receive, it's inevitable that their wines will command eye-popping prices. Millions of people in the world not only associate legendary names like Lafite or Romanée Conti with the highest quality in wine, but also wish they could have a sip of their wine. Unfortunately, the number of bottles available for sale can never catch up with their fame. This drives the price up to stratospheric levels, which only garners them more attention. Once again, all the attention is given to the wines we never get to drink.

Plots and Deceptions

The reasons why wine producers pay so much attention to location are understandable, but for ordinary consumers the way the names of locations are used to market wine can sometimes seem downright misleading. In the popular imagination, which many producers shrewdly exploit, all wines are made at the vineyard by the vineyard owner. In fact, winemaking and vineyard management are each challenging professions and it's rare that the talent for both resides in a single person. If it is, that person faces the added challenges of finance and management, and isn't likely to produce large quantities of wine. As a result, the brands most readily available to consumers are those made by volume producers, who grow their grapes in multiple locations or source them from others, sometimes growing little of their own. In these cases it is the skill of the winemaker more than the specific location where the grapes are grown that has the most influence on the final product, but you typically hear little about it.

The ability of winemakers to consistently create a sizeable quantity of wine with a consistently recognizable taste is an art that is rarely appreciated by the consumer, partly because so many in the wine industry have been reluctant to admit how much they rely on technical talent. Great winemakers often defer to the quality of the grapes as the most important factor in making a great wine and speak of the benefits of "not getting in the way." But their humility in the face of nature is only a sign of their considerable wisdom. Don't be fooled into thinking that they don't have as much to do with the success of the final product as the location where the grapes are grown.

Since the image of being a prestigious domain wine is worth real money to the folks who produce wine in volume, it's not surprising that they may be inclined to take advantage of this in their marketing and labeling, and thus compound the popular misconception that all wines are somehow handcrafted at an estate where the grapes are grown. Together with the fact that most restaurant wine lists and retail establishments tend to organize their wines by country or region, this helps to reinforce the impression that location is the best starting point for learning about wine and that the association of the wine with a prestigious location is the most important factor in determining how satisfied you'll be with the wine you choose. This can be quite misleading.

Loco Labeling

Although many areas have established regulatory systems intended to identify with a degree of precision the geographic origin of a wine, these are not always as helpful as they should be. Remember that for every rule about wine there is at least one exception, usually more. This makes the effort to mandate standards for labeling wine a bureaucratic minefield, one that only the French (who've only been working seriously on it for less than 200 years) have navigated with much success.

For the average consumer, even French wine labels are confusing. In most of France, for example, the wines from the very best locations are classified as *"Grand Cru"* and the second best locations are classified as *"Premier Cru,"* even though *"premier"* means "first." In France's best-known wine region of Bordeaux, however, the top locations are classified as *"Premier Grand Cru,"* with the emphasis on *premier cru* or "first growth." Then, of course, Bordeaux itself has an exception in the commune of St. Émilion, which has its own classification system that puts the emphasis back on *"Grand Cru."* The proof of the authenticity of French wine, you see, is that there are exceptions to the exceptions, even in the labeling.

In some countries, like Germany, the rules have a long and controversial history and the system can seem almost as if it was designed to mislead rather than inform. Here the authorities go to great lengths to ensure that the precise bottling date is on the label, but aren't quite so precise about the exact vineyard.

Other countries like the United States have had the luxury of starting with a relatively clean slate. The process is in its infancy, but so far the labeling effort in the United States seems just as confusing and susceptible to petty squabbling as it is everywhere else. As in France, a great deal of attention goes into identifying "viticultural areas." Much less attention is given to labeling by grape variety even though consumers in the United States focus more on varietal designations than geographic sub-regions. The labeling laws permit wines to be named after only the principal grape variety used to make the wine, while the names of other included varieties that can have a major impact on its taste are permitted to be undisclosed. As a result, many Americans drink blended wines thinking that they are made from a single variety.

Thus far, the poorly paid public servants in charge of the U.S. labeling laws seem to have only a limited comprehension of the dynamics of the wine trade. They have concluded, for example, that leaving the "an" out of the word "Santa" would be sufficient to allow consumers to distinguish between certain American and Chilean wines. To Americans, this might seem simply a pragmatic solution to a small dilemma, an uncharacteristic recognition that the average consumer treats the official viticultural area as largely irrelevant. To the Chileans, it might have seemed a bit loco, in hindsight perhaps even a bit of a gift.

In the United States and elsewhere, even though a producer trucks in wine from hundreds of miles away, it may be permitted, depending on the local laws and how strictly they are enforced, to sell the wine as "estate bottled" if it's bottled at a winery located on a vineyard that it owns. Also, many new wineries give their wines names that sound vaguely similar to the names of prestigious wine estates or even regions far removed from the location of their vineyard (a practice not unknown to upstart producers even in France, where the laws are lenient about a producer using a family name even if it might confuse the unwary consumer). Meanwhile, many of the legendary producers in France and Italy have begun ventures in Spain, California, Oregon, Chile and Argentina, to which they lend their expertise and the names of their famous estates. That leads to domain names showing up in unexpected places.

Ineffective regulation is only one aspect of the problem. Even in areas where the rules are reasonably logical and strict, there is always the problem of unscrupulous operators at every level in the supply chain. Adulteration and fraudulent labeling further complicate the task of trying to understand wine from the ground up and add to the confusion of the average consumer.

Location Overload

Deceptive labeling, fraud and ineffective regulation aren't the main problems the average consumer has in focusing on specific locations, however. The main problem is that there are just too many of them. Within every wine-growing region there are areas that produce very different wines and within each of these areas there are communities with distinctive microclimates. Even within each of those communities there can be several of those tiny plots that get all the attention. So in the traditional geographic introduction to wine, we might first be introduced to the eminent region of Bordeaux and then to one of its sub-regions, such as Pauillac. After a detailed explanation of the microclimates within Pauillac, we are told that one of the most prestigious wines from that area comes from the domain of Château Lafite-Rothschild.

There's plenty of information here, but none of it helps you predict what the wines will taste like. Never mind that you can't afford to drink Lafite regularly or perhaps ever; nobody has described what the wines from Pauillac or even Bordeaux taste like, nor could they do it easily because there is so much variation. So knowing the name of a region and which of its domains is the most prestigious doesn't really help you choose a better wine to go with your noodle soup, does it? In fact, there are simply too many locations to keep track of even if you want to make a profession out of it.

Learning to distinguish between the different tastes of all the wines made from just the principal vineyards in a single region takes a great deal of training and intimate familiarity with the region, yet many people begin their wine education by trying to do just that. By contrast, it takes relatively little time to learn the differences between the major grape varieties. It isn't a snap, but I can show you how to make it much easier and have fun in the process.

Although there are many grape varieties, only a few are used to make the vast majority of the wines available to consumers on a regular basis, and most of these are used, to a greater or lesser degree, in every region. If you begin your effort to understand wine by trying to remember all the different locations in which wine is made, you'll have thousands of names to remember. Although the specifics of soil, exposure and growing conditions typically used to describe a particular wine-growing location can influence the taste of a wine in subtle ways, the taste characteristics most important to you in selecting wines for various occasions don't depend on these specifics. They are related to the basic structure of wine (which you now know), the principal characteristics of the grape varieties used to make it and the style of wine the winemaker produces with them.

In Appendix B, I've listed the major grape varieties used to make wine and organized them into five groups. If you understand the characteristics common to these groups, you will know most of what you need to make successful wine selections. Many of these characteristics are created by the particular mix of acids produced from the grapes, so it's helpful to learn how the most significant of these acids affect a particular wine.

Variety and Flavor

You're already familiar with the role that tartaric and tannic acids play in giving a wine body and texture. As you start to sort through the various grape varieties, it will help you to understand the role that a few other acid groups play in giving a wine flavor. Although it can play a significant role in determining body and texture, a grape variety's most significant contribution to a wine comes in the form of flavors, particularly the characteristic fruit flavors that are associated with various wines.

The roles played by acids associated with citrus fruits, such as citric acid, ascorbic acid (vitamin C) and their by-products, are quite different from tartaric acid. While tartaric acid gives wines a straightforward and durable sourness, citric acid provides noticeable fruity flavors like lemons, limes and grapefruit. These give wine a keen edge, but break down fairly quickly. Dry wines made with grape varieties exhibiting these flavors, such as Riesling and Pinot Grigio, are usually crisp, delicately flavored white wines made for fairly early drinking.

When warmed and exposed to certain bacteria, citric acid breaks down naturally to produce acetic acid, which is the primary component of vinegar. Combined with alcohol during fermentation it also produces ethyl acetate. Winemakers work hard to control the amount of acetic acid and ethyl acetate because they're volatile and can enter a gaseous phase at room temperature, which spoils the aroma of a wine. When professionals refer to a wine as overly acidic, they're referring to harsh volatile acids that result from the breakdown of citric acid.

Citric acid also gradually breaks down into a number of other acids that ultimately degenerate into diacetyl, a compound that can give wines, especially white wines, an "oxidized" taste. Sulfur dioxide treatments and filtration, the controls winemakers use to prevent this, aren't popular with many wine drinkers because residual sulfur sometimes produces headaches and excessive filtration can dramatically strip flavors out of the wine. Citric acid is consequently the diva of wine acids. It can deliver thrilling flavors, but is hard to control.

Another important acid in wines is malic acid. Its name is derived from the Latin words for apple and harsh, so it's not surprising that wines that are high in malic acid exhibit green apple flavors and a harsh, biting edge. While not so quick to degenerate as citric acid, malic acid can be broken down by certain bacteria in the later stages of fermentation. The result is lactic acid, the principal acid in milk, so the breakdown of malic acid into lactic acid makes a wine seem buttery and softer. For many red wines, this is a desirable trait, but for many white wines (Chardonnay being a notable exception), the taste and smell of lactic acid can ruin the delicate citrus flavors. Think of drinking a mixture of buttermilk and lemonade.

Although it's not necessary to be able to pick out the various flavors and other tastes in a wine according to the acids that create them, it is useful to understand how the crystalline structure of tartaric acid establishes a stable, sour base for the taste of wine, how tannic acid affects its texture and how other acids give it less stable fruit tastes that can break down and change over time in more or less pleasant ways. This is the basic framework for understanding both the larger aspects of varietal taste and its subtlest nuances.

How to Own a Grape Variety

Your savvy as wine consumer will grow much more quickly if you begin by learning to understand the characteristics of the major grape varieties than it will if you begin by trying to understand all the details of soil and microclimate at the world's major wine domains. In Appendix B, I give descriptions of twenty-one of the most commonly used grape varieties and describe how they influence the taste of the wines made from them. Even though that's far fewer than the number of leading domains many introductory wine books might expect you to become familiar with, it still might seem to be a bit of a chore to become thoroughly familiar with all of them. Rest assured, this Appendix isn't intended for that purpose.

Appendix B is intended only as a brief introduction to the most common varieties used to make wines throughout the world today. It notes the regions they originated in, the regions they're most closely associated with today and their similarities and genetic relationships to other varieties. As you should expect, I've concentrated on the taste characteristics that most people associate with these varieties. By now, I'm confident that you've learned to judge wines for yourself first and then match up your impressions with the consensus view.

Although the descriptions in Appendix B are economical and brief, you don't need to read all of them in order to select the varieties most likely to appeal to you. Alternatively, you can choose the varieties that show up most often across from the foods you like to eat in Appendix C, which describes some very broad food and wine pairings. Use these appendices to narrow down your initial focus to one or two varieties. Once you've become familiar with them, you'll want to move on to others, but at the outset, it's prudent not to be too ambitious. It's going to take time to master the characteristics of all these different varieties, but there will be plenty of different wines for you to drink even if you are concentrating on one or two.

After doing a few comparative tastings with the wines made from the varietals you've selected to start with, it won't be difficult to recognize the various characteristics they contribute to the wines you drink. It helps to do the comparisons properly, however. Many introductory wine-tasting courses begin by doing side-by-side comparisons of different varietals. This can be useful to show you the differences between their tastes, but it can be misleading as well. You may assume that every attribute of the wine given to you as an example of a particular variety is an attribute of that variety, when many of them are likely to be traits reflecting soil characteristics, climatic influences, weather conditions or the stylistic choices of the winemaker.

To truly understand the essence of a grape variety, its inherent characteristics need to be distinguished from those created by conditions under which the grapes were grown and the wine was made. In my experience, it's easier to learn these inherent characteristics when you concentrate first on wines made exclusively from a single variety. By keeping the varietal constant, it's easier to recognize the impacts of soil, climate and winemaking style, and see how they interact with varietal characteristics.

It's by comparing one variety to another that you to begin to understand what makes a varietal unique. But you have to own the taste of at least one variety before you can make comparisons. And you own the taste of a variety only when you understand it well enough to be able to subtract out the elements that are independent of its varietal characteristics. To learn to do this, it's necessary to taste wines from a single varietal that are made under various conditions and in different styles. Then you can learn what makes it unique by comparing it to other varietals. In that process you'll be learning how to identify the other varietals as well.

Searching for Flavors

Unfortunately, the task of finding wines made from a particular variety isn't always as easy as it should be. Wines in many European countries are identified only by place name, so you can't tell which wines are made from which varieties by looking at the labels. In other areas, the variety will be listed on the label, but the label may be misleading, because the law may only require the producer to list the *predominant* grape variety the wine is made from. Significant amounts of other varietals may be included in the mix, without being disclosed, to improve its color, make up for various deficiencies or make it more palatable to consumers more accustomed to other varieties.

Sometimes just adding small amounts of wine made from other varieties can dramatically alter the taste of a wine. In fact, the ability of small amounts of certain varietals to impart a dominant taste to a wine is part of the reason that many wines are blends of wines made from different varieties. So be careful. If the label doesn't say that the wine is one hundred percent from a certain variety, there is a good chance that there are complicating elements in the bottle. It can help to do a bit of homework, but the practice of doctoring wines isn't something people who sell wine are anxious to talk about, so be sure you're getting reliable information.

Another difficulty you will face as you begin to familiarize yourself with the taste of different varietal wines is that the references wine professionals make to the various flavors in different wines aren't always precisely what you might first expect. It's important to realize that these references to fruits, herbs, spices and other tastes are only approximations, because they refer to *tastes in wine* that others have come to associate with the foods referred to, rather the characteristic tastes you might normally associate with those foods themselves. So when experienced wine drinkers say a wine has a hazelnut taste, they're sensing a taste in the wine that reminds them more of what hazelnuts add to a dish than anything else they're familiar with, not that it tastes exactly like a hazelnut.

Because wine writers are so accustomed to using shorthand references that most experienced wine drinkers will recognize, they may fail to mention whether a fruit taste they are referring to is to the unripe, ripe or dried form of the fruit. Sometimes they also refer to tastes that people in one part of the world might be familiar with, but others aren't. This is why British wine writers refer to black currants, while American wine writers refer to Cassis, since black currants themselves are rare in North America, while the liqueur made from them is more common. To compound matters even further, wine writers often like to display their familiarity with exotic foods as well as exotic wines. This can all be quite confusing for the uninitiated.

Wine writers talk about flavors in wine the way we talk about the man in the moon, so perhaps it's not surprising that their descriptions seem a bit spacey to many people. When we try to assimilate the complicated and changing face of the moon into a recognizable pattern, it's natural for us to think of a face, because we see faces everyday and some of the common elements in faces, such as their overall roundness and patterns of light and shadow, are reprised in the image of the moon. Even though the image isn't precisely like a face, or particularly masculine, we get it when we hear others refer to the man in the moon, and have a sense that they see the same image we have in mind when we refer to it.

As you learn to pick out the essential characteristics of a specific grape variety, you'll begin to feel more comfortable that you understand what wine writers and others say about the taste of a wine and you'll start to feel your wine-tasting abilities reaching a state of full maturity. Learning to identify varietal flavors will help you develop an even deeper perspective on the characteristics in wines that vary from region to region and you'll be able to appreciate even more keenly how the taste of the wine is influenced by the style of wine that the producer is seeking to create. You'll also notice that, while many of the elements of style are primarily associated with particular wine regions, winemakers in other regions can use them as well, creating divergent styles within styles and raging controversies among wine lovers.

The Elements of Style

As you begin to appreciate how a good winemaker can accentuate the differences between major grape varieties, or even stand them on their heads, you'll gain a deeper understanding of the elements of winemaking style. Winemakers use many tools to modify or enhance the inherent characteristics of their wines. As a result, there are almost as many wine styles as there are winemakers, but the basic elements of style aren't difficult to recognize and these are the ones that have the greatest impact on the taste of the wine.

The style of a wine results from specific decisions made during the winemaking process. Understanding several key variables in this process can help you comprehend the basic elements of style that many wines share.

One of the first decisions made by the winemaker is the amount of contact to allow between the juice in the grapes and their skins and stems, because the flavors that the winemaker is trying to bring out can often be overwhelmed by the tannins and other substances caused by that contact. In most white wines, for example, this contact is usually minimized. What can give body and structure to these wines are minerals brought up from the deep reaches of the soil by mature roots, sometimes extending down hundreds of feet. When you see old vines being advertised on the label, look for the taste to be enhanced by mineral flavors as well as by the more concentrated tastes that the naturally limited yields of old vines produce.

Although they can sometimes be simply a mixture of red and white wines, most rosés are wines produced from red grapes in the same way white wines are produced from white grapes. The winemaker uses grapes that are less ripe and limits the time the juice spends in contact with the skins and stems, creating a wine that is lighter in color and lower in alcohol. Because of these qualities, rosés tend to be favorites for luncheons or afternoon drinking. Many people prefer sweeter rosés made from riper grapes, such as the blush zinfandels with their legions of young American fans or the somewhat less sweet rosés from Portugal that are reputed to be a favorite of HRH Queen Elizabeth II. Other rosés, particularly those from southern France, are drier wines, made with restrained fruit so their herbal qualities can be more in evidence.

When red grape varieties are used to make a classic red wine, the bolder flavors from these varieties can blend well with the tannins produced by contact with the skins and stems. Often fermentation is allowed to begin inside the grapes before they are crushed, or partially crushed grapes may be allowed to sit in a cool vat for an extended period before the final pressing is done and the juice is drained off to make the wine. These techniques can bring out bold tastes in the wines, making them feel heavier and more mouth-filling.

Tannic Tension

We've already discussed how tannins play a particularly dramatic role in changing the feeling in our mouth because they contain molecules that bind with the proteins in saliva and make the mouth increasingly sensitive to touch as we drink wines that contain them. Together with higher levels of alcohol, they also combat bacteria and allow the winemaker to produce wines that can be aged to develop special textures, flavors and scents. An elevated level of acidity can also turn the bite of a high-alcohol wine into a bracing grip and introduce flavors that suggest green peppers, grasses, eucalyptus and herbs, such as mint.

In the hottest wine-growing areas, the grape varieties have flavors that will stand up to even more alcohol. To me these wines "light up," showing hints of tobacco, tar and black pepper. As you might expect, winemakers who live in these warmer areas tend to spend more time outdoors and do more open-pit cooking and barbecuing. The wines seem designed to match.

When a vineyard is capable of producing grapes with vibrant and intense flavors, the winemaker may choose to boost and enhance the tannins in the wine even further by aging it in wood for a period of time. The tannins in the wood can blend harmoniously with the tannins in the wine and further help to preserve it while it ages. They impart mouth-filling flavors, like vanilla, and can also give the wine a fresher, cleaner aroma, reminiscent of cedar.

Not all wines are meant to age, however, and the use of wood can be overdone, especially with white wines. Because the flavors in white wines are more delicate, winemakers need to take special care to select varieties of wood and techniques for using them that don't overwhelm the flavors of the wine. When California wines first gained recognition as having world-class potential and earning power, various producers tested the ability of their Chardonnays to produce wines with staying power. It's not surprising that initially a rash of "over-oaked" wines found their way to market, and then the phenomenon gradually receded.

The Old Age Question

The degree to which a wine is made to age or be consumed early is a fundamental factor in determining the style of wine that a winemaker creates. When a wine is made to age, more intense flavors must be extracted from the grapes. These intense flavors are necessary because otherwise the high levels of alcohol and acid necessary for the aging process to proceed successfully will overwhelm them.

To some extent, the issue of longevity underlies the differences between the styles of wine that are considered old-world and new-world. As discussed earlier, however, a key element in the development of new-world wine styles has been the extension of grape culture into areas that require irrigation and the development of strains that place less emphasis on earthy, mineral flavors.

Regardless of where they are producing them, when winemakers look to enhance the earthy tones in their wines they cannot simply amplify the fruit in their wines to balance out the alcohol and acidity. As a result, they will use special fermentation techniques that soften the acids in the wine and use strict production controls that allow them to produce lower-alcohol wines that can still age well. These techniques can help to produce wines of singular character that showcase the characteristics of the soil and climate in their area regardless of whether they are in a new-world wine region.

Some traditional producers complain that all new-world-style wines are simply attention-getting wines being made by younger producers. Though they might be biased, there can be some truth to this. Even in a long-established wine region, an upstart producer is likely to have younger vines and more new oak barrels, so it's not surprising that they would promote the fruitiness of their wines and the amount of new oak used to produce the wine. After a few years, the barrels won't be so new and the roots of the vines will have penetrated deeper in the soil, picking up more earthiness and minerality. At that point, you might notice the wines take on a more old-world style, as well as a shift in emphasis in how the wines are promoted.

Whether the winemaker's decisions are the result of design or necessity, they have a significant effect on the taste of a wine. In particular, they will affect the degree to which a wine seems balanced. By controlling the length of fermentation, the winemaker can influence both the amount of alcohol in the wine and its residual sweetness. By controlling skin contact and the exposure of the wine to wood, as well other techniques, winemakers can influence the amount and complexion of a wine's acidity. All these factors affect the body and texture of a wine and provide a structure that can enhance and enliven both the varietal flavors and the tastes contributed by the soil.

The Value of Similarities

As you can see, it's essential to be able to recognize the more evident elements of taste contributed by the grape varieties and winemaking style in order to really understand the unique qualities contributed by *terroir*. In the next few chapters, I'll help you understand more about how you can use your understanding of these basic elements to help you drink your wines at the right time, in the right place and with the right food. This will improve your chances of enjoying them much more than getting to know all of the locations where they are made.

You may be determined to develop an appreciation of the finer points of all the world's great domains. Even so, you will need to develop an understanding of the ways they are similar to other wines first, so their unique qualities stand out more clearly. The unique qualities are what provide the largely unpredictable pleasures we thrill to on the rare occasions when we have the opportunity to enjoy these wines. The similarities are what we can connect with on a day-to-day basis.

If your memory is much better than mine, you *could* con-ceivably commit to memory all many details that are cataloged and freely available about the soil, microclimate, vintages, ownership and history for hundreds of prestigious estates in all the far-flung corners of the world, but it will take much more time and effort than it's worth. It will take you so long, in fact, that in the process, you'll end up missing out on many good wines you might have enjoyed even more than the prestigious wines you're studying about.

Hallowed Names

Because many consumers are finding it easier and more reliable to differentiate wines by varietal characteristics, producers are increasingly recognizing that naming wines after places can limit their marketability. In new-world wine regions in particular, whose locations have less global recognition than wines produced in Western Europe, producers market wines to the export market almost exclusively based on varietal designations. Place of origin is usually mentioned as well, but given much less prominence.

Where place names are important today, it's usually because the place is associated with a particularly celebrated style of wine. A wine made from Chardonnay may be referred to as "White Burgundy," "Chablis" or, if sparkling, "Champagne," because the areas they come from are well recognized for producing a particularly sought-after style of wine made from Chardonnay grapes. Similarly, red wines made from Pinot Noir might be referred to with increasing geographic specificity as "Red Burgundy," "Gevrey-Chambertin" or "Romanée-Conti," because these locations are well recognized for producing extraordinary wines made from Pinot Noir.

Other situations where special locations have iconic identification with a particular variety include "Rhine" and "Mosel" wines for Riesling; "Barolo" and "Barbaresco" for Nebbiolo; "Sancerre" and "Pouilly-Fumé" for Sauvignon Blanc; Beaujolais for Gamay; "Chinon" and "Bourgueil" for Cabernet Franc; "Napa Valley" for Cabernet Sauvignon; and, in a somewhat nascent way, "Argentine" for Malbec. Of course there are the inevitable exceptions, such as in Italy, where "Super-Tuscan" is a term identified with wines made with Cabernet Sauvignon and Merlot, rather than the region's most celebrated variety, Sangiovese, and the regional wines (which have increasingly become associated with Sangiovese) are called Chianti, except in the standout communities of Montepulciano, where the local Sangiovese clone takes the name of the town, and Montalcino, where the local clone is named "Brunello" after the color of the grape. No wonder Italian wines have a reputation for being the most confusing of all!

Blending In

In other areas, it's not the ability to create a style of wine particularly suited to a single variety that draws attention to the name of a particular place, but the ability to create a legendary style of wine using a blend of different varieties. For example, in the Bordeaux region in France, Merlot is the dominant grape and is used almost exclusively in a majority of the wines produced in the region. The wines in the Médoc area of the Bordeaux region, however, are famous for blending Merlot with Cabernet Sauvignon, Cabernet Franc and other varieties, so that wines produced in other regions that blend these varieties are called "Bordeaux blends."

In Spain, where it plays a workmanlike role similar to that of Merlot in Bordeaux, Garnacha is blended with Tempranillo to produce the wines that made the Rioja region famous. Similarly, in France's Rhône Valley, distinctive wines made by blending Garnacha (Grenache in French) with Syrah and other varieties have made the communities of Châteauneuf-du-Pape and Hermitage famous. In California, winemakers emulating the styles of these wines proudly called themselves "Rhône Rangers."

With blended wines, Italy once again distinguishes itself by its flexible rules. Thirty years ago, "Chianti" referred to wines made by blending wines made from Sangiovese with wines from numerous different varieties. The winemaker had considerable flexibility in the wines chosen for the blend, but was required to include a certain percentage of white wine made from the Trebianno varietal. Today, however, white wines have been banned from the Chianti mix and the wines are increasingly becoming focused on Sangiovese. This is not altogether surprising. As growing and winemaking methods in a given area evolve, there is an inevitable tendency to concentrate on the varieties that prove to be most popular. Grape varieties used simply to stretch these varieties, rather than contribute something ineffable to the blend, fall by the wayside. In the case of Chianti, as the blend has become more focused on Sangiovese (which has been favorably affected by climate change in the region), its reputation has been burnished and the name has become associated with an exemplary style of wine made from the Sangiovese grape.

Whether resulting from their skill at blending wines or working with a single varietal, winemakers appreciate that complexity is the characteristic that makes the wines associated with the legendary vineyards in their area stand out. Wines take on cult status when producers are able to work with their unique microclimates to transcend the one-dimensional profile that might otherwise characterize their single varietal wines. Similarly, many blends started out as a practical response to the vagaries of weather, employing difficult to grow or late-ripening grapes to add something special to wines made from more pedestrian but reliable varieties when the weather permitted. But certain blends have persisted because of their ability to deliver more complex flavors and a broader range of combinations with food.

The famous place names in wine, therefore, do owe their special status to soil and climate, but often in a much more subtle and indirect way than many people imagine. In many cases, one of the rarest phenomena of all, effective government regulation, has also played a major role. By requiring producers to adhere to standards that promoted noteworthy characteristics in the wines from a particular region, regulators have in some cases standardized both the quality and the characteristic style of the wines from the region sufficiently to attract a broad market and ensure that the product that reaches the consumers is consistent with what they expect.

Composing the Image

Once you understand the basic structure of wine, the different tastes of the major grape varieties and the climatic and stylistic factors that influence those tastes, you can begin to compose an image in your mind of the various wines that come from the world's various regions. As you start to recognize these regional differences, you'll also start to identify the regions most likely to produce the wines that best match your taste preferences and budget. If you have an old-world palate and find wines made from the Sangiovese grape pleasing, you can begin your exploration of the wine world in Tuscany. If you have a new-world palate and find you like Shiraz, learn a little bit more about the wine and food scene in Australia. Ultimately, you may be able to travel to the region, meet the producers and see the vineyards. Nothing fixes the characteristics of the wines from a certain region in your mind more than a visit.

I recommend that you begin your exploration of wine regions by focusing on a single region that produces wines you already enjoy. You're likely to find the foods produced in that region and the local style of cuisine agreeable as well. Look for an affordable wine made exclusively from one of the principal grape varieties the region is known for. When you find an affordable one you really enjoy, buy a case of it and try it out with different foods. After you've worked through a few bottles in the case you should become sufficiently familiar with it to try some of the other wines from the region that are made from the same grape variety. Notice the similarities and differences in taste and price and see if they make sense to you. Learn who the best known-producers in the region are, decide for yourself which ones you like best and compare prices. (This is particularly important if you're unlucky enough to start with a region whose wines tend to be more expensive.)

Changing Focus

By developing a thorough familiarity with one grape variety and region at a time, you'll give yourself concrete points of reference to use as you expand your knowledge. If you have strong preferences for the region you started with, it will probably make sense for you to begin expanding your knowledge using wines from the same region that are made with different grape varieties. You can then move on to blended wines that use these varieties.

If, on the other hand, your preference is more oriented toward the grape variety than the region you started with, you can progress to wines made from the same variety in other regions. As long as you use wines you've become thoroughly familiar with as a touchstone for a logical series of step-by-step comparisons, you'll progress at a surprisingly rapid pace. You'll soon gain a natural appreciation of how varietal, stylistic and regional factors play a role in determining which wines you will like best and which you will prefer to avoid.

As you move from varietal to varietal and region to region, your ability to make distinctions among wines should grow in a series of concentric circles. For example, if you start your search with Chardonnay as the varietal constant, you should find the differences between new-world and old-world styles the easiest to make because new-world style Chardonnay is generally more full-bodied than old-world style Chardonnay. This will divide your first circle into two parts. Next, you'll notice the rather obvious difference that the use of oak contributes, giving wines a more pronounced edge because of the texture contributed by the tannins in the oak. Since both new-world and old-world style Chardonnays include oaked and un-oaked versions, the next circle of understanding will be divided into four parts, two on the bottom and two on the top.

As you move out from the most broadly shared characteristics to the more variable ones, your next circle might divide the various quadrants into broad fruit categories, like citric vs. tropical fruits, and these might be further divided in the next circle into specific fruits like green apples, lemons, limes, pineapples, and so forth. Finally, you will get to characteristics like minerality and spiciness that are more location-specific.

Many people engaged in the formal study of wine find it useful to use aroma and taste "wheels" that chart these increasingly refined characteristics for various wines. You may find it helpful to refer to a diagram like this too, or to try and make one for yourself, but it's not really necessary. What's far more important is to use the process of building a mental image to train yourself to analyze wines in a systematic way as you drink them. As you gradually begin to identify increasingly subtle characteristics for each grape variety, you'll inevitably make changes and adjustments that would require you to redraw the diagram many times. Meanwhile, the image in your head will adjust flexibly, moving up, down and around in exactly the way that's needed in order to develop the best tasting instincts. You'll also find that, as you become more familiar with the process of analysis, your train of thought will move much more quickly than your eyes can sort through a diagram. Eventually, the mental process of breaking down categories will simply become an instinctive part of your ability to recognize a wine, and you'll start to focus instantly on the unique qualities of each specific wine: the ones experts tend to focus on, but that you found difficult to recognize until you had a context to put them in.

As you learn to place wines in context and tease out the subtler characteristics of the wines you like best, it will become easier for you to recognize the wines you'll enjoy most when you see them. Since you'll be more attuned to their subtle charms, you'll obviously want to avoid drinking them at the wrong time or pairing them with the wrong food. The information in the next few chapters will help you learn how to use wine to bring out the best in food, people and other aspects of your life. As you become skilled at using this knowledge, you'll inevitably broaden your field of view to include wines made from more and more varieties and regions. With this broader view, you'll be more aware of the possibilities available to you when you select and consume wine and be better able to take full advantage of them.

As you learn to place wines in context, your appreciation of your own taste will also evolve and you're likely to become more adventuresome. You may find that the wines you truly love best are entirely different from those you first began to learn about. But you're more likely to find that what you learn about each new varietal and area brings you an even better understanding of the wines you already thought you knew. Sometimes, the old flames burn brighter even as you follow a new star.

Bringing Out the Details

Once all the more obvious things that should guide your choice of a wine become second nature to you, you may find yourself alive to those small territorial differences that express themselves uniquely in the wine from a particular estate or commune. But you should do this only if you feel specially rewarded for the effort when you pull the cork. If you aren't there yet, don't worry about it. You don't need to own the mountain to enjoy the view.

Soil and weather are complex systems that humans struggle to understand on a day-to-day basis. Talented winemakers will opportunistically take advantage of their variability to create something surprising and unique from each vineyard and each vintage. With sufficient time and attention, these qualities will become increasingly apparent to you.

As the famous empiricist David Hume observed in his 1757 essay, *Of the Standard of Taste,* the deepest appreciation of anything as subjective as taste is best acquired through the practical knowledge that comes from experience. He noted how it's easier, when we first observe a thing of beauty, to judge the overall effect than to distinguish the individual qualities (objects) that produce it:

> But allow him to acquire experience in those ob-
> jects, his feeling becomes more exact and nice: He not
> only perceives the beauties and defects of each part, but
> marks the distinguishing species of each quality, and
> assigns it suitable praise or blame. A clear and distinct
> sentiment attends him through the whole survey of the

> objects; and he discerns that very degree and kind of
> approbation or displeasure, which each part is naturally
> fitted to produce.... In a word, the same dexterity, which
> practice gives to the execution of any work, is also ac-
> quired by the same means in the judging of it.

As you become increasingly familiar with the larger elements in the taste of different wines, the smaller distinctions will emerge and the beauty of *terroir* will become apparent to you. Eventually you'll find that *terroir* is about the little things that make a big difference once the big things have been properly attended to. It's an expression, not just of the land, but also of the place: encompassing the soil, the climate, the local winemaking techniques and the cultural traditions of the people who tend the fields and make the wine. In a region where both winemakers and wine drinkers are steeped in the notion of *terroir*, you'll not only taste the soil in the wine, but find it reprised in the taste of the local foods. You'll become curious about how the wine is treated as it makes its way from the vineyard to you and, learning the effort involved, you'll appreciate the wine even more.

As they learn more about wine, most wine lovers go through several stages: in the first they learn what wines they like. In the second, they learn how to match those wines with the foods they eat. In the final, enduring stage, they begin to incorporate wine into the social fabric of their lives and enjoy participating in the ongoing flow of information between producers and consumers that has shaped the world of wine for centuries. It is this ancient dialectic that is largely responsible for the extraordinary quality and diversity of the wines available to us today. By participating in it, you connect yourself with a formerly hidden dimension and your wine experiences begin to resonate with both the deeply reassuring cycles and wildly unpredictable anomalies of nature.

Henri Jayer, the legendary Burgundian winemaker, used to say that each wine he made was "a message in a bottle," an expression of the soil, the vintage, his art and his feelings about his place in the world at large. When you taste a wine and can see the vineyard and hear the words of the winemaker, you're no longer just buying bottles of wine and you're certainly buying more than just property. You've entered into a great and timeless conversation and are sharing a special kind of love.

Poor Timing

How to drink wine at the right time

The vintage mark on a wine bottle, which shows the year in which the grapes were harvested, is a tangible reminder of the intimate relationship between wine and time. The success of the vintage in every wine region is closely watched. Charts assigning numerical scores to the vintages of various regions are updated annually. Books are sometimes written just about the good and great vintage years in a particular wine region.

While vintage deserves much of the attention it gets, other more important timing issues are routinely ignored. Most of these have to do with things that can happen after the harvest and many are things you have more control over than the weather in a given year. Poor timing can ruin your experience right up to the moment you pour your wine into the glass. So a proper understanding of the relationship between wine and time is essential.

Vintage Confusion

The importance of vintage is often misunderstood. The proof is in the prices. A top wine from a highly touted Burgundy vintage can command four times the price of the same wine from a lesser vintage. Similar disparities exist between the prices of the most sought-after wines from Bordeaux and other well-known wine regions.

Does this make sense? It can if you're interested in prestige. The impact of scarcity and name recognition on prices applies to vintages as well as locations and producers. A wine from a celebrated location and producer is even more prestigious if it comes from a rare vintage.

But such large differences in the prices of vintage are not as apparent with lesser-known wines. Since the essential difference between a good harvest and a bad harvest is the weather, that doesn't make a lot of sense. A good year will provide a longer window for picking the grapes at their peak, so a good year is a year when even the lesser wines shine. If prices were oriented toward quality rather than prestige, there would be less disparity between the prices of the top wines in good and bad years and more disparity between the prices of the lesser-known wines. That it's the reverse shows how often the issue of vintages is misunderstood.

When a wine expert describes a good year, you may hear about the flowering conditions in the spring, the average summer temperature or the luminosity of the sky. But these are the curlicues on the cake. The basic element of a good year is perfect conditions for the harvest. If there's excessive rainfall during the harvest, all the little niceties of the growing season will be trumped.

Prestigious producers can minimize the effects of poor harvest conditions by commanding the resources to pick their grapes more quickly on the few days when conditions are ideal, while other producers wait in line for the men and machines necessary to complete their harvest. Top producers also own the vineyard locations with the best drainage and exposure to the sun—those least likely to be adversely affected by bad weather. Thus, the importance of the best harvests, as can always be seen on the happy faces of the vineyard workers, is that *everyone* gets to pick their grapes under ideal conditions. The grapes produced by an ideal harvest don't need to be lavished with attention and expensive treatments in order to make great wine. That's why winemakers say wine "makes itself" in a great year; all they need to do is not get in the way. You can get very good, even great wines, from all but the worst producers in the good years and the prices of the wines made by less well-known producers won't skyrocket the way the prices of wines from the great domains do.

Great domains will typically make extraordinary wines even in bad years, however. They have a reputation to protect and wouldn't think of producing anything less, despite the extra expense involved. This gift is generally appreciated by only the savviest consumers.

Excellent values can also be found in the wines from average vintages. It's not uncommon for every vintage to be surrounded by a certain amount of hype when it is released and it may take a while before it dies down and a consensus emerges as to whether the vintage is a truly great one or just another also-ran. At that point, the wines will languish on the shelves and retailers and restaurants will want to clear them out to make space for a newer vintage that is being showered with hopeful praise. This is often an opportunity for shrewd buyers. They may have already tasted the wine and found it quite satisfactory. Here again, time and a bit of confidence in your own ability to taste can be richly rewarded.

As you can see, it pays to learn about vintages. This is not so you can then buy the best wines from the best vintages, as many people assume. Instead, you should buy the less expensive wines in the good years, the more expensive wines in the bad years and the moderately priced wines from an average year only after all the hype dies down and it's recognized as such. It's only when you properly understand how to use what you learn about good and bad vintages strategically that you can get better value by knowing the differences between good and bad years. Then you can take advantage of the opportunity to drink some extraordinary wines when they aren't getting the attention they deserve.

Time Traveling

You can also get better value from any wine if you pay attention to its age, regardless of the vintage. Timing is critically important, not only in the winemaking process, but also in the decisions you make about storing and serving wine. If you don't understand the importance of these decisions, you'll do yourself a disservice much more often than you will by not choosing the most ballyhooed vintages. It's far more important to drink wines at the proper time than it is to drink "proper" wines.

The voyage that wine takes from vineyard to table is a journey through time as well as space. It's particularly important to understand the relationship between time and temperature when it comes to wine, because most of the time it pays to take your time and be cool. Even though a certain number of sunny, warm days are necessary to ripen grapes, cool breezes and mists can help extend the growing season and the window for the harvest by helping to maintain firmness and acidity levels. This allows time for more complex flavors to develop in the grapes and prevent them from building up so much sugar that the fermentation process gets out of control. Grapes can just get cooked over a long, hot, stifling summer and the resulting wines will lose some of their freshness and appeal.

Cooler temperatures are also useful during the winemaking process, which is why there has been increasing use of temperature-controlled fermentation vats. A winemaker may have to warm up his juice a bit to get fermentation started, but for the most part cooler fermentation temperatures slow things down and give the wine more time to develop unusual flavors and scents.

In the winery, timing decisions play many important roles in determining the style of wine that's produced, including the most fundamental style choice, whether to produce an early-drinking wine or a wine made for aging. White wines, which are usually made to drink within a year or two of their release, lack many of the ingredients that time provides for wines that are made to last. The grapes are harvested earlier and the juice is usually left in contact with the stems and skins for a shorter period than with red wines. It's rare for them to be put aside in wood casks for any significant period of time, so they are ready to go to market sooner. If you tend to prefer whites to reds, you're lucky. They should be, and for the most part are, cheaper, because they take less time to produce.

There are also many red wines that are made for early drinking. In fact, it's a trend. Many wines that have traditionally been made to reach their peak in ten to twenty years are now being made so they reach their peak much earlier. This change in time frame is a controversial subject. "Traditionalists" argue that people who produce wines that are more approachable at an early age are just profiteering by avoiding costs and taking advantage of consumers who have been browbeaten into accepting earlier-maturing wines by self-serving commercial interests. "Modernists" claim that the traditionalists are just stuck in a rut and won't admit that many consumers prefer the style of an earlier-drinking wine. Meanwhile many wine consumers seem to enjoy having the choice, or at least having something to argue about.

Taking the Time to Make Great Wine

While the choice of a producer to make an early-drinking style of wine may be controversial, the benefits provided by time to a wine that's been made to age are not. Wines made to be aged benefit from extra time in many ways: extra flavor and color are provided by extended skin contact at the beginning of the winemaking process and more complex acids result from the time spent in wood casks. But time's greatest gift is the magical change that occurs when these wines are simply left alone in a cool, dark place for a long time. Grape variety, *terroir* and differences in production play an important role in determining which wines will age and how long, but the winemaker's decision to commit to the time and resulting expense of a wine that will last is fundamental.

Young wines, with their crispness and fruitiness, should be an important part of anyone's wine-drinking repertoire. In addition to pairing better with certain foods, they generally chill better and can brighten up a hot afternoon or an overheated room. Wines made to age, however, whether red or white, offer an entirely different set of tastes and textures. The breakdown of tannins and other acids makes them smoother and easier to digest, while time brings out flavors that become more subtle and intriguing as they get older.

Many of the world's most exciting wines are spectacularly different when given a decade or more of proper storage. Their evolution during this process is a curious one that isn't as well understood as it should be. While they can taste fruity and bracing when young, they go through an extended middle age, when they will taste decidedly funky, before they emerge as mature wines of great sophistication. Far too often, they're consumed before they're able to reveal their greatest talents.

Unfortunately, it's not an easy task to get these wines to their peak, and events that happen long before the wines are put down for storage can make the entire effort worthless. Any good wine importer will tell you that the way a wine is shipped and stored can have a major effect on its ability to age properly, because it can get "cooked" by being confined in a hot container or warehouse or left out on a sunny loading dock. Good importers, shippers, distributors and retailers will take special measures, such as using temperature-controlled shipping containers and air-conditioned warehouses, to prevent this. Sadly, this is still the exception, rather than the rule.

Since many consumers don't have proper facilities for storage or much experience drinking well-aged wines, they drink the wines long before their time, impressed by the prestige of the brand or relying on ratings and vintage rankings they don't understand. Here the flaws created by improper shipment and storage are less evident, because the wines are either being consumed so early that the evidence of their mistreatment hasn't had time to become obvious, or a bit later, when they're in their funky period and taste a bit off anyway.

The sad fact is that it takes time for the effects of mistreatment to be recognizable by the average consumer and some members of the supply chain are tempted by this to cut costs when they ship and store wines. In fact, given the evident willingness of consumers to drink age-worthy wines too early, it's quite remarkable that so many major participants in the industry resist this temptation. If the people you buy your wines from make a special effort to avoid these problems, try to remember to express your gratitude.

The Burdens and Benefits of Cellaring

For the consumer, it can require a significant investment to create the facilities for proper storage, and the cost of maintaining an inventory of aging wines is also a significant consideration. Even if only one-third of the wines you drink each year are expected to be aged an average ten or more years, the cost of acquiring these wines will add significantly to your wine budget during the decade or more it takes you to build up to a level where the inflows and outflows are evenly matched.

The task of storing wines while they age is largely left to the consumer. This probably has ancient origins, since growers typically didn't have facilities where these wines could be properly stored and their wealthy customers did. Today, since most people still have trouble finding the space for a wine cellar, it would be easier for the producers rather than consumers to store wine until it was ready to drink. Yet producers still outsource this task (and the risk of bottles going bad). Understandably, for many people, the considerable investment of money, space and time required to properly age wines doesn't seem worth it.

Historically, fine restaurants have taken on the challenges and risks of storing wines. Unfortunately, even though more and more restaurants are featuring their wines, the bottles on their lists are also getting younger and younger. Meanwhile, it's becoming increasingly difficult to find older wines for sale anywhere but at auction. These auctions sell only the most prestigious wines to the most serious and well-heeled wine collectors. So, if you want to get well-aged wine for a reasonable price, you still have to do it yourself.

Having a wine cellar provides many benefits beyond the ability to age wines. Having suitable storage space can allow you to purchase even early-drinking wines more cheaply, by the case or at special sales, and hold them until needed. It also helps immeasurably to have a selection of wines readily available for a special occasion or just to pair with whatever you feel like eating on a given day. If you have the space and the budget to put away several years' worth of wine, however, the opportunity to properly age your wines is the main reason to have a cellar.

Some of my friends use commercial units that can maintain the proper temperature in a kitchen, garage or other area where constructing a cellar might not be feasible. These units generally have limited capacity, but additional modules can be added as the cellar builds. I also have friends who live in smaller homes or apartments and make use of the commercial wine-storage facilities. For younger fans of older wines, this can be a useful way to build up an inventory, which can be transferred to an in-house cellar at a future time. While these are typically more expensive ways to maintain a cellar than sectioning off a cool part of your home, they can sometimes provide much higher quality storage space than you can afford to create there.

However you find a way to properly cellar your age-worthy wines, it's certain to pay off in the long run, as long as you're careful to select and manage the wines in it. This isn't as easy as it might seem, so I hope you have better luck with it than I did. It's taken me over twenty years to learn how to make the best use of the wine cellar in my home. Constructing the proper space was only the beginning of the process; understanding how to use it was equally important.

Deep Misconceptions

When I first began to put down wines, a few misconceptions prevented me from making the best use of my cellar. The first was thinking of the widely recommended storage temperature of 11°C (about 55°F) as more of an average than a strict upper limit. I wrongly assumed that the main effect of having the cellar reach higher temperatures for limited periods of time would be that the wines would mature more quickly. Instead, I found that only a day or two at higher temperatures was enough to flatten out wines that had aged gracefully for many years. Since the processes that deteriorate a wine can move very rapidly at higher temperatures, I had to learn to become extremely vigilant about avoiding them by taking precautions against power failures and equipment malfunctions while I was away for extended periods.

Recently, I've had the opportunity to taste wines that were stored at temperatures much lower than the recommended level for long periods of time. Somehow, the processes that give wines the ethereal qualities of age seem to work even better, if more slowly, at cooler temperatures short of freezing. The consensus view seems to have set the recommended temperature for a cellar with the average middle-aged wine collector, rather than the wine, in mind. It's been set close to the upper limit of what is safe because otherwise we might not live long enough to appreciate our beautifully aged wines.

I can't necessarily recommend keeping a cellar below the recommended level, because the time it took my wines to age, even at that temperature, tested my patience. Having a cellar made it possible for me to buy wines that needed to age, but they didn't always get a fair chance. I was constantly tempted to try the wines that were aging when I ran out of other wines to drink or just to satisfy my curiosity about how they were coming along. Only when I reached the last few bottles did I appreciate how foolishly I had squandered the rest of a case. I had to learn to better manage my cellar and make "defensive" acquisitions of early-drinking wines in order to be sure I wasn't tempted to drink my other wines too soon.

Even with these precautions, it took time for me to discover how to best match the capabilities of my cellar to my needs. Although I generally buy six or more bottles of the wines I put away for the long haul, it's still disappointing to open one of them too early. Critics' notes and even reports from the very active wine underground can be helpful, but don't always relate to what I experience. For me it's usually safer to keep a bottle a bit past its peak than to open it a bit before it, even though that's well within the drinking window recommended by others.

It also took me a long time to develop a feel for the different wines I normally consumed over the course of an average year and maintain the right quantity of each type, so that I wouldn't end up with too much of one and too little of another. The trick, of course, is to make additions that would approximate my normal consumption pattern for each type of wine over the course of a year and leave me with a cellar as well balanced at the end of the year as it should have been when I started. But it's not as simple as simply replacing what you consume, since different events occur each year. My interests and tastes also evolve from year to year and each wine has a slightly different aging profile. Even now, I end up accumulating too much of one type of wine and not enough of another (although, since the surplus bottles have now become my "defensive" wines, that's not such a bad problem to have).

When I do run short of the wines I'd like to have in my cellar, the simple expedient of buying more of the things I ran out of doesn't really plug the gaps. In fact, it can create further imbalances. I've gradually developed an algorithm that tries to take into account all the different variables that affect my consumption patterns. These patterns keep evolving, though, so I do envy those who can afford to overstock. A well-aged wine isn't difficult to give away. Think of all the friends you can make.

Adolescent Awkwardness

Since wines will taste funky during the bulk of the aging process, it's not possible to cut your losses by drinking them up if your find yourself running out of space. Many people don't have space to keep an adequate supply of well-aged wines for everyday drinking. Unless you limit your consumption of these wines to special occasions, you'll need to build a cellar of some size, so it's important to properly assess your needs and manage your expectations before you start. If you don't have the proper amount of space, you'll end up waiting a long time and only be able to drink a few bottles every so often, which may not be worth the effort. Even if you have large cellar, if you don't have the time to manage it properly, you'll end up with imbalances that can make much of the effort to store the wine a waste.

For anyone who has a wine cellar, there will inevitably be some ups and downs. I've occasionally discovered bad lots of wine after storing them for years in my cellar, but the number has been far less than I expected. Far more often, I've found a bottle that has been held far beyond when it was supposed to be at its peak. These rarely disappoint; more often they are sublime.

Now that I've learned how to avoid careless retailers and pay careful attention to drinking windows, the older wines that I pull from my cellar seem to be in much better condition than the older wines I've occasionally been served in restaurants. They're much less expensive as well.

While I resent being offered a wine list littered with bottles of age-worthy wines that are too young to drink, I rarely drink older wines in restaurants. Given the challenges of storage and the apparent willingness of consumers to drink wines well before their time, well-aged wines appear only rarely on restaurant wine lists, usually at prices I can't afford. The only way to satisfy my yearning for them is to buy them when they're first released and try to be patient.

Decanting Demystified

If you have the space, money and patience to cellar your wines, you'll be well rewarded. Just make sure the effort doesn't go to waste by a few moments of neglect when the time comes to drink them. Older wines are much more fragile than younger wines. The time they spend at your table is a small fraction of the time it takes them to get there, but it can be the most perilous. With all the effort that it takes to cellar a wine, don't let it be abused at the last minute.

When most people think of old wines, they automatically think of decanting: the process of transferring the wine from the bottle to another receptacle before it's served. The image of an elderly gentleman delicately pouring wine from a dusty old bottle into an elaborate carafe (usually while holding a napkin around the neck) has been an icon of fine wine service for centuries. This is quite different, however, from the typical contemporary usage.

Because it's become so difficult to find older wines on the market, today decanting is most often used as a way to try to accelerate the aging process for younger wines. For speed and thoroughness, an aerating device of some kind is sometimes used as well. While it's not really a substitute for proper aging, vigorous exposure to air can take the edge off a tight, tannic young red wine and even help enhance the flavor of some young white wines.

Once a bottle is open, the amount of air the wine absorbs before you drink it can be critical to your level of enjoyment. Most younger wines will "open up" and give off more aroma and flavor if they are given time to absorb air and warm up a bit after they are released from the bottle. You can easily experiment with this at home and get a feel for how important it is. Just pour a youthful wine and taste it. Notice whether the aroma is noticeable and how much flavor it delivers on the first sip. Then let it sit in the glass for a while and swirl it about a bit. This will aerate it and may also warm it up a bit.

As it sits in the glass, the bottle or a decanter, most people find the taste of a good young wine continuing to improve for much longer than they expect. In fact, they often find that the wine seems best long after they might normally have finished the whole bottle. Once aware of the issue, they're more likely to request that a wine be decanted before they drink it or will at least give it some time to breathe in the bottle and the glass before drinking it.

Originally, however, decanting had nothing to do with aeration. It was used to avoid the sediment that's stirred up when a bottle is tilted back and forth multiple times as wine is poured into a number of glasses one after another. The idea is to leave most of the sediment behind in the bottle, and pour the clearer wine from the decanter into the glasses. Since the wine had already been properly aged, no vigorous aeration was necessary...or necessarily desired.

With older wines, pouring wine into a decanter can be a bit of a trade-off. On the one hand, the older a wine is, the more gritty sediment it can have. On the other hand, mature wines can be fragile. Aging a wine always involves some level of deterioration, which is accelerated when the wine is exposed to air.

An older wine can be at its peak for less than an hour after it's poured. So it's generally a good idea to drink it fairly promptly after it's poured. If it still seems a bit ahead of its prime, it can sit for a while in the decanter. But if it's at its peak, it shouldn't be left to sit too long. You might not even want to risk decanting it. By the time you finish that, it could have lost much of the delicate charm bestowed on it by patient aging. Always take the time to taste a sample from the bottle before you decide to decant it.

Finding the Right Time

The significance of the year in which a wine was made varies as time progresses. In the end, knowing a wine's vintage is more important for what it tells you about how to serve and drink the wine than it is for what it tells you about how good the wines from that year are relative to other years. The weather during the growing season determines the levels of sugar, acidity and flavor in the grapes and the character of the wine that the winemaker fashions in response. This determines the appropriate drinking window for the wine, which in turn affects decisions about when and how to serve the wine. As you build your understanding of these relationships, you'll be able to better manage the crucial final minutes before you drink the wine.

Remember that, as wine breathes, it lives. Next time you sit down with a bottle of wine, take some time to notice how the wine matures in the bottle and the glass. You may be able to literally watch it as it sheds its youthful awkwardness and emerges into graceful maturity or as it loses its youthful charm and settles into a boring equilibrium. When you're drinking a wine early in the drinking window (or often now even before it reaches that window), make sure it's decanted or given sufficient time to breathe after it's first poured. For wines near the end of the window, be vigilant to avoid too much exposure to air or you may find the wine collapsing right in front of your nose. By giving a few moments of attention to this issue each time you drink wine, you can quickly fine-tune your awareness of how exposure to air affects different wines at different times. Meanwhile, the next time you're in a restaurant and you see someone making an inordinate show of decanting a bottle, swirling the wine around and putting it aside "to breathe," you can be sure that there is at least one wine on the list that's a bit too young to drink.

New Dimensions

Thinking about the aging process and the effects of temperature and air will add important new dimensions to your understanding of wine. It can help you enjoy the wines you love at their best. If you have the resources to start a cellar, it can also provide a pleasant pastime as you plan and manage it, and even more pleasant results when you drink and share the wines that you've aged.

If you don't have the resources to create a proper cellar, don't waste your precious resources buying wines that are made to age. Learn more about wines made for earlier consumption. There are sure to be many that you'll readily enjoy. Eventually, I hope you'll find opportunities to learn about the increasingly rare pleasure of a well-aged wine. Don't pass them up!

There are a number of stratagems you can employ to gain access to well-aged wines, even if you don't have a cellar. You may find a wine group in your area that supports a communal cellar or you can start one with some of your friends. These groups typically use the excellent facilities provided by commercial wine storage warehouses, which today have on-line resources available to allow customers to manage their cellars from home.

Maybe you're lucky enough to have a restaurant or wine bar in your area that actually serves wines that are more than a few years old at reasonable prices. If so, patronize them. What they are doing isn't easy.

Most of all, if you know someone who does have a good cellar, figure out what you can bring to the party so you can share in the bounty. Cellar owners invariably accumulate more than they need and I don't know anyone with a good cellar who likes to drink alone. This is another way time works in our favor.

Adding the dimension of time to your understanding of wine will help you appreciate the dynamics that determine not just what a wine is, but how it's best used. Learning the virtues of older wines will help you appreciate the situations that younger wines handle better, while knowing when to serve a wine, and how it changes as it's served, will help you conserve its talents so you can appreciate them more. As your understanding of the many relationships between wine and time deepens, you'll feel them harmonize and intertwine. You'll begin to hear all the various instruments that wine can play in the symphony of life and see many new ways it can improve both your everyday experiences and your most special moments.

Learning about time's complex relationship with the wines you drink is deeply rewarding and endlessly fascinating. As with everything else, time is relative when it comes to wine: sometimes patience is rewarded, sometimes you have to seize the moment. As you become more sensitive to the various nuances of wine and time, you'll see the connections between your past, present and future wines more clearly and the perspective will allow you to organize and execute your wine experiences with more finesse. By being able to pick not just the right wine, but the best time to drink it, you'll find new rhythms to step to as you advance in time with your wine.

Mismatching

How to choose the right wine

Whenever you're selecting a wine, even if it's a modest one, there is a match to be made. With all the many choices available today, the process of matching can seem rather daunting, but it needn't be. To do it well, all that's required is to keep wines in their proper context by avoiding a few problem areas. It's an application, rather than an extension of what we've been doing all along. As attentive trial and error makes you better and better at predicting how different wines will taste in various circumstances, you can let your natural instincts guide you through the final frontier of wine enjoyment.

There was a time when food and wine choices were limited and the choices most readily available worked fairly well together. Today, however, there's much more diversity in what we can choose, how it's prepared and where we consume it. Serendipity and romance have their place, but you still have to be selective. The opportunity to make a better match has increased, but your chances of making a mistake have increased even more.

Poor wine pairings are the most common mistake I see. I shouldn't be surprised, since it took me so long to learn how to make good ones myself. Yet good pairings aren't difficult to make and I've found that a modest wine properly paired with food can give me as much pleasure as drinking an expensive bottle by itself. So I'm still a bit startled to see so many people who love wine mess up their pairings.

As I look back with the clear vision of hindsight, I see that good pairings were an essential part of those memorable experiences where I first became aware of wine's ability to captivate me. I don't think I'm unique. Ask most wine devotees about a memorable bottle of wine and they'll often tell you as much about the overall experience and the food as they do about the wine.

My wine epiphany was in the dining room of a gracious old hotel. We had come in for a late dessert after a long flight. The kindly and dignified sommelier suggested a Spätlese from the Mosel that simply seemed supercharged with Bananas Foster and Cherries Jubilee. Several months later, attending a small celebration at a private club, I was served a Puligny Montrachet with Quenelles of Pike for a first course and felt I would rather drink more of that wine than finish the rest of the meal. Not too long after that, on a beautiful May evening on the Bay, I found my rack of lamb perfectly complemented by a Napa Valley Cabernet Sauvignon. It wasn't just that these wines and foods made nice combinations; the taste of each seemed enhanced in turn by the last taste of the other.

In each of these cases I walked away with the label from the wine bottle, naively thinking that the trick was simply to get more wines like these. I wasn't totally oblivious to the great settings, friends and foods that made these wines shine. I just knew it was the wine that got my attention.

So I bought some books, began to study up on wines and started to acquire wines that had a reputation for being special. When I paired them poorly, I initially persuaded myself that a great wine should only be enjoyed by itself. Somehow, it was easier for me to think of some wines as too good to match than to accept the fact that I was ignorant. As I've since learned, what often makes a wine great is its suitability for a certain type of occasion or its ability to pair well with a broad range of foods. Drinking it by itself is a bit like drinking it alone. It's pleasurable, but not as much fun. It feels as if even the wine is lonely.

When I make pairings today, I think of that lonely bottle and try to choose wines that have the best chance to feel welcome and be themselves in the situations I'm placing them in. Once I eliminate the awkward wines, the ones that remain are usually quite good at rising to the occasion. If I don't see something that seems obvious, I'm happy to give something else a chance to surprise me.

Now that you understand the most important factors that influence your enjoyment of a wine, you can use that understanding to keep wines in their comfort zone. With a little practice and common sense, you can dramatically reduce the odds of picking the wrong wine by simply eliminating the worst choices from consideration first, so you can concentrate your attention on those that remain. To eliminate inappropriate wines most effectively, however, it's important to be fully aware of all the factors at work. Though it's customary to think of pairings in terms of food and wine, there are other factors that can be critical. Sometimes food isn't a factor at all, or it will play only a supporting role, and many pairings that make sense in isolation are inappropriate in a broader context. This makes it important to consider all the factors that have a bearing on your decisions from the outset, so let's start our exploration of pairing by looking at some important considerations other than food.

Making a Sparkling Choice

To give each pairing a fair chance to be an adventure, you have to be careful not to get lost before you start out. It's good to take some bearings. Whether you're in a wine shop, a restaurant, or ordering a wine online, it pays to stop and think about where you're going to be and how you're going to feel when you drink it.

Suppose you're being asked to choose the wine for a special occasion like a graduation or a wedding. It's customary on such occasions to think of Champagne. Practical considerations might dictate that various sparkling wine alternatives should be considered, but food generally plays a subservient role on such occasions. It's useful to understand why.

What helps Champagnes and other sparkling wines set the right mood for a celebration is the sparkle. Part of that is visual, of course—the little bubbles just seem to be doing a lively dance—but the bubbles have another important role. They are the by-products of carbonation, which causes alcohol to be absorbed into the bloodstream much more quickly. So when waiters arrive with trays of sparkling wine the party really lights up!

Another factor that makes sparkling wine a good match for a celebration is the fact that it can be served cold. This can be an important benefit when a room gets crowded and stuffy, or when you're celebrating outside on a warm, humid day. The predisposition of the people drinking the wine (the kind of mood they want to be in) and the setting (the surroundings in which the wine will be served) are dominant factors in choosing wine for a celebration. These two factors are always useful considerations whenever you're choosing a wine and will help you narrow down your choices in a meaningful way. Eliminating wines that don't fit the setting and the mood will prevent you from making many of the most obvious pairing mistakes.

Setting the Stage

Whether you're buying a glass of wine to drink right away or a bottle to put away in your cellar, it's important to consider the setting in which you're expecting to drink the wine and the mood you expect to be in or are trying to create. Understanding how these factors influence your enjoyment of different wines is an important first step in learning how to make successful pairings.

Let's consider that you've just spent a rather warm afternoon at a sporting event. You enter a restaurant and appreciate the refreshing coolness of the air conditioning. You probably feel hot and thirsty now, but the air conditioning could make you feel chilly fairly soon. It's probably not the right time to order an expensive bottle of champagne.

Expensive wine is hardly ever a logical choice when you're hot and thirsty. You'll be inclined to quaff it in order to satisfy your need for hydration, which is a mistake because the alcohol in the wine evaporates quickly through your skin and is dehydrating. Drinking wines too quickly can leave you feeling flushed and overheated, exactly the opposite of what you require. So, it's better to take your time reading the wine list and have a few glasses of water while you do.

Even when you buy wine for future consumption it's useful to think about the setting in which you expect to consume it. If you're buying ahead for the next weekend, think about the weather report, where you expect to be and who might be joining you. That can narrow down your choices a bit and maybe even help you understand why some of those bins at the front of the shop are marked down. The wine in them may be nearing the point where they don't make sense for the season any more.

If you're stocking your cellar, the wines you're buying to put away are likely to be for special occasions, especially if you have limited storage area. Think about the types of special occasions you celebrate in your home, what dishes might be featured and what kind of wines work best with them. You'll also want to think about how your home is configured. If you have a large dining room and like to entertain larger groups you'll need to buy more, or perhaps larger, bottles to put away. If you have limited space inside your home and often do your entertaining outside, you may want to concentrate on lighter wines that can be more refreshing in warm weather or denser, spicier wines that will stand up to barbecue.

While you're contemplating the scenery and other surroundings that make up the stage on which your wine will perform, you'll also want to think about the audience: you and the others you'll share the wine with. How receptive they are to the character of a wine ultimately depends on who they are and how they feel. In a drama in which the members of the audience play a leading role, their age, gender and other personal characteristics are essential considerations.

Sex, Shape and Age

For many people, wine helps to create a romantic mood and plays a part in the enjoyment of sex. Few seem to realize that our sex also affects our enjoyment of wine. Women tend to enjoy lighter wines with lower alcohol because their bodies metabolize less alcohol in their stomachs. As a result, more alcohol passes on to their intestines where it's picked up by the bloodstream. (Lower levels of the estrogen-sensitive enzyme alcohol dehydrogenase seem to account for this.)

Body weight is also a factor that affects blood alcohol levels. As women tend to be smaller than men, it's sensible for them to drink lower-alcohol wines. Wine drinking isn't boxing, so there's no particular glory in learning to take a punch like a heavyweight. More likely, you'll end up on the ropes. If you're a heavier person, however, don't be surprised if drinking a lightweight wine makes you feel like a bit of a sissy. You'll probably feel more comfortable in your own weight class.

As we age, our palates become less sensitive to certain tastes and others stand out more. At the same time our range of experience tends to become wider and our receptiveness to various tastes can become more diverse. Young wine drinkers are likely to prefer sweeter, fruitier, less-expensive wines, since they appeal to both their palate and their pocketbook; older ones tend to be more comfortable with drier wines, with low acidity, since they tend to avoid eating spicy or greasy foods that are harder to digest.

While our tastes can change in predictable ways over time, they are also fickle and can shift from time to time, in less predictable ways. We can be influenced by trends among our friends and in the media or just get tired of what used to be exciting, but now just seems like the same old, same old. When buying wines to put away you should keep your fickle palate in mind. A wine that seems to be all the rage right now might be a has-been when it's ready to drink. You should also think about your own age. You might be buying wines that only your children will enjoy.

Serious Business

While people often think of wine when they are planning a celebration or a romantic evening, there are many other situations in which a judicious choice of wine is necessary to create a proper mood. For a business meeting, you'll want to think carefully about when or even whether wine should be served. The alcohol content will certainly be a consideration, as well as the messages your selection conveys about your sophistication, spending habits and regard for your guests. How a business associate chooses and handles wine is often observed carefully.

Even when you're alone or with close friends, there are issues of personality and mood that you should consider in selecting the wines you drink. There are times to dance and make noise and there are times to chill out and be mellow. A fruity, low-alcohol wine might help you keep your footing and your cool while you mambo; a spicy, complex wine with more alcohol might be just the right thing if you're settling down in your deck chair to watch the sunset on a lazy afternoon.

Whenever you get ready to select a bottle of wine, take stock of the surrounding circumstances before you begin to consider your choices. What is the weather going to be and how might it affect you and your companions? Who will be drinking the wine and what do you know about what they like? Where and when will you be drinking the wines and what will you be doing afterward? These factors are critical when the occasion is oriented around an event or has a goal beyond just sharing a meal. Even for an occasion where a meal is the main event, they can help orient your thinking and make sure the wine you choose is a better fit. A perfect match is a wine fit for the occasion, the surroundings and the people, as well as the food.

Matching Wines with Food

I often wonder why so many people have good taste in matching clothes and bad taste in pairing wines. They don't seem to have nearly as much trouble putting together a decent outfit to wear for a particular occasion as they do picking a wine to go with a nice meal. One explanation could be that people get dressed every day, but drink wine only occasionally. Yet there are many people who drink wine every day and still have more trouble finding a wine to complement their meal than they have finding a pair of shoes to match their outfit. This is odd because the process of matching textures and colors in clothes and matching textures and flavors in wine and food is so similar. We simply need to learn what complements and contrasts in a way that's pleasing rather than distracting and throw in a subtle dash of something extra if we want to be super-stylish.

There are many professionals and dedicated amateurs who have raised the process of matching food and wine to an art form. They regularly fashion transcendent pairings that can render you speechless and bring tears to your eyes. On some serendipitous occasions such innately beautiful pairings happen accidentally, but more often they are the result of careful collaboration between professionals: such as a sommelier with a prodigious knowledge of wine and a good understanding of food, and a chef with a prodigious knowledge of food and a good understanding of wine. Creating these spectacular pairings typically requires not only a depth of knowledge most of us don't have, but a certain amount of trial and error, hard work and inspired intuition.

We can't afford to put so much trouble and effort into ordinary pairings and we don't need to. Fortunately, making decent and even very good matches isn't that difficult. Gasps and tears of joy aren't the objective of our everyday pairings. Rather, it's to avoid awkward clashes between incompatible elements. This will keep the combination in a zone where things work reasonably well together—the zone where serendipity can happen, but isn't necessarily expected.

The Basics

To make good, rather than just workable, everyday combinations doesn't take much more effort than we make when we choose the clothes we wear. We need only learn to be careful about a few things: the first is how to deal with certain troublesome foods, the ones you shouldn't try to pair any more than you'd wear a dinner jacket or cocktail dress to the office or a fly-fishing outfit on the rugby pitch. The second is to avoid clashes between the weight and texture of the food and wine, the way you wouldn't wear a heavy woolen shirt under a seersucker jacket. The last is to respect dominant elements and keep accessories under control, the way you take that big, floppy hat off when the horse race is over.

Two basic factors require us to pay attention to food and wine parings. The first is that all wines have qualities that enhance the enjoyment of foods. In addition to moistening the palate when the foods we eat make it dry, wine also contains enzymes that stimulate the appetite and aid the digestion. Like fruit juices, it contains acids that can clear the palate and freshen it for the next bite of food, but the fruit flavors in wine are more muted and less likely to compete with or overwhelm the food. Since these factors are common to all wines, they allow most of them to enhance the taste of almost any food.

Most good table wines, and even most mediocre ones, have the ability to complement a broad range of foods. We instinctively acknowledge this when we order a glass of house red or white with our hamburger or seafood salad. The wine might taste a bit thin and scrawny in the face of greasy or creamy foods, but more often than not the food benefits from the combination...and we're not expecting the wine to taste that good anyway.

Once you've made the easy decision to add wine to a meal, however, you'll need address the second basic factor involved in wine and food pairings: foods have no common characteristics that make all wines taste better. Despite all the effort wines make to be friendly to them, foods are selective about the wines they work best with, and some just plain mess up the taste of many wines. Thus, while wine usually enhances food, food often impairs our ability to enjoy wine, which ruins two things: the wine and the meal.

Fussy Foods

The ability of most wines to go reasonably well with a broad range of foods may be one reason wine pairing doesn't get the attention it deserves. Another may be the general tendency to consider it the responsibility of wine drinkers to select wines to match the foods that are available. As a result, the person preparing the food may not think to avoid, or at least place in proper perspective, foods that can interfere with the enjoyment of the wine.

You can dramatically increase the chance that what you drink matches what you eat, and avoid confusion over what goes with what, by learning how to deal with a few troublesome foods. You may, in fact, have had many great pairings in the past, but didn't know it because these fussy foods interfered with them.

Several very common foods are particularly troublesome with wine. Runny egg yolks, chocolate and soft cheeses tend to coat the palate and diminish our ability to taste wine. Green asparagus and members of the cabbage family, which include broccoli, brussels sprouts, cauliflower and turnips, contain sulfur compounds that bring out vegetal characteristics and can interfere with delicate wine aromas by giving off a slightly skunky smell. This is why people go to the trouble to grow white asparagus, serve red cabbage or mix their sprouts with carrots and caramelized onions. Artichokes contain cynarin, which can confuse your palate so you perceive flavors that aren't really there. (It usually creates a sense of sweetness where there isn't any, but for some people the reaction is reversed and artichokes make wine taste peculiarly bitter.)

Shellfish and fish like mackerel, haddock and cod can contain iodine, which makes them problematic with tannic red wines, since the interaction between the iodine and the tannins creates a metallic taste in both the wine and the fish. The acetic acid from vinegar in salad dressing, and other foods like pickles and sauerkraut, occurs naturally in many wines, but not in the concentrations that are contained in vinegar. In wine, a detectable vinegary taste is usually considered a flaw, which is why the French take their salad after the main course and the Italians leave the vinegar out of the salad dressing.

The wide range of textures and flavors in vegetables can also call for special handling with wine. These can range from the rich, dense sweetness of corn to the sharp sting of peppery greens such as arugula and radicchio. Even though acidity can be more noticeable in white wines, it may not be sufficient to stand up to raw vegetables. Sometimes a splash of lemon or lime can brighten the acidity of the dish and make the wine pairing work better. Just as the fruit flavors of red wines are more muted than those of the fruits whose qualities they reprise, so their herbal qualities tend to be more muted than those in vegetables. Red wines tend to pair better with vegetables that have been cooked, perhaps with a bit of salt.

Challenging Cheeses

With a wide assortment of cheeses and wines to choose from, Europeans have identified many fabulous wine and cheese combinations, but that doesn't mean wine and cheese match each other routinely or that the wine doesn't suffer a bit in the exchange. The French, who call a meal without wine breakfast, are very careful with their cheese and wine. They tend to use cheese sparingly in the early stages of a meal, unless they have a fairly good idea what wine will be served and have a cheese that goes particularly well with it.

There is a saying among wine professionals: "Buy on apples, sell on cheese." The light citrus flavor of the apples stimulates the taste buds and helps a buyer pick up flavor nuances, but cheese coats the palate and can disguise flaws in the wine. Implicit in the slogan is the expectation that people are unaware of how cheese interferes with the ability to taste a wine.

This helps explain why the "wine and cheese party" has become an entertainment staple for charities. For a large gathering, a charity would be profligate to spend lavishly on good wine. By serving some gooey cheeses, flaws that might exist in more inexpensive wines can be covered up.

With a little skill or luck, however, knowledgeable guests at a wine and cheese party can often put together a respectable pairing. Most wines will enhance the taste of hard cheeses, although you'll find it's usually best to stick with a dry white wine for a soft creamy cheese, unless they're moldy, when a sweeter white is necessary to avoid too sharp a taste. Sweet wines also work best when matching salty cheeses, as they can make tannic wines taste particularly bitter (this can also be countered with honey). Cheeses made from the tangy milk of goats or sheep will work best with lively younger reds. In fact, many of the most popular wines are known for pairing well with a popular and ubiquitous cheese: Merlot and Camembert; Chardonnay and Brie; Cabernet Sauvignon and Manchego; Sauvignon Blanc and a creamy goat cheese. These wines and cheeses are relatively easy to find and can make classic pairings in their own right.

The fact that there are so many wonderful pairings of specific cheeses and wines is undoubtedly why so many people have an incorrect impression that wine and cheese are a friendly combination in general. There are classic pairings for other wine-unfriendly foods as well. Chocolate desserts with rosé Champagne, or another sparkling rosé such as Bugey-Cerdon, are a staple of the romantic novel and an offering that almost no one will turn down. If you like the herbal, grassy flavors of Sauvignon Blanc, green asparagus can enhance them; even artichokes will pair with Grüner Veltliner.

Learning that certain foods can be both unfriendly to wine and successfully paired is an important insight into wine and food pairing. It not just a matter of looking for matches, but also a matter of understanding what gets in the way and what the overall objective of your pairing is. If you like artichokes, you'll learn to drink drier wines with them. If you pay attention, you'll also learn to avoid drinking tannic red wines with oily fishes. With a bit of practice, you can learn to juggle your way around most of these problem foods so they don't interfere with your basic wine pairings. Then, since you'll have conquered the toughest challenge, you can relax and have fun; the rest will be easy.

Body and Texture in Food

There are tactile sensations we experience when we eat food, such as weight, hardness, fibrousness, slipperiness and chewiness that are related to the way we experience body and texture in a wine. These qualities are so familiar to us that we don't commonly think about them and, since they're shared by many foods with different flavors, we don't normally associate them with taste. They play a major role, however, in the interplay between food and wine.

Just as we can use our natural ability to sense whether a wine is light-, medium- or full-bodied, we can sense the tactile differences between foods like fish, poultry and red meat and can instinctively appreciate how lighter foods will be overwhelmed by a full-bodied wine, while heavier foods will make a lighter wine taste thin and scrawny. This is where an understanding of the tactile qualities of various wines is most valuable, since we can use it to match the textures of various foods.

Where either delicate or heavy textures dominate a meal, careful matching is required in order to keep either the wine or the food from becoming too dominant. Many raw, steamed or lightly grilled fish and vegetable dishes, or dishes consisting principally of rice, have lighter textures that can easily be overpowered by a full-bodied wine. A light-bodied wine will be lower in alcohol, glycerin and tannin, have less impact on your palate and preserve your ability to enjoy the delicate tastes of these foods.

Fatty meats and oily fishes, such as beef, lamb, herring and mackerel, and dishes with creamy sauces or heavy gravy, have a heavier feel and coat the palate. They call out for full-bodied wines with higher levels of acid and alcohol. These can aggressively scrape the palate and help reprise the unctuousness of the first bite of food throughout the meal, so we don't become so quickly satiated that the meal becomes boring. When these foods have a fibrous chewiness, it can be complemented by the raspy texture of a wine with higher levels of tannin.

For the broad range of dishes that are neither light nor heavy, a light-bodied wine will feel insipid and a full-bodied wine will be too dominant, but almost any medium-bodied wine will work and you'll have a certain amount of leeway to choose between textures that complement or contrast. Many dishes made from poultry, veal, pork and most cooked fish and vegetables fall into this middle category. Here, the overall texture of the dish is likely to depend on how it's prepared. If prepared simply and cooked so the fats and oils drain out, these medium-bodied foods can pair with a lighter-bodied wine. On the other hand, when they are incorporated into richer dishes, using ingredients such as bacon or cheese, or served with gravies or cream sauces, the wine should be more full-bodied.

In this middle range, slightly contrasting the weight and texture of a dish to maintain an overall balance is usually more successful than reprising them, since the additive effect of heavy on heavy can be overwhelming and light on light can leave you feeling unsatisfied. Just remember that a successful pairing interferes with neither the food nor the wine; so don't lay on the contrast so heavily that it becomes overwhelming.

Although it's not a perfect system, I like to think of wines as having "knife edge" qualities. Lighter-bodied foods like clear soups and fresh or flaky fish and salads either slip off the edge of a knife or need a knife with a very sharp, straight edge, such as a salad knife, to cut them neatly. These often go with crisp, lighter-bodied wines with citrusy tastes. Creamy soups, fish, and meats like poultry and pork will either stick to a knife when it's dipped in them or can be cut easily by a normal dinner knife. These foods are in the broad middle range of foods that make good combinations with medium-bodied wines. I associate full- bodied wines with high levels of tannins with the rough edge of a serrated knife. These wines work best with meats that are fibrous and fatty, the ones for which a steak knife is handy.

Major and Minor Notes

Most dishes tend to be structured around a dominant taste. In some cases, food can also be prepared to serve as a background for the dominant taste of a great wine. When intense tastes compete for dominance, the qualities that make them great can be lost, which is a great waste of both money and pleasure. This has led to the frequently repeated caution (not a rule, but a reminder): "Don't upstage the star!"

When you're choosing a wine to pair with food, stop and think about the dominant flavor as well as the weight and texture of the dishes you're pairing with the wine. This is not necessarily what the recipe or the menu identifies as the main ingredient. In some dishes, the main ingredient, like a type of fish or meat, is simply a base on which to build a dish that showcases another more dominant element, like an herb, spice or rich sauce. In that case, it's a safe bet that a wine that complements or reprises this element will be a successful match.

A dominant taste may not be a single flavor. Some tastes are combinations and contrasts between flavors. As any good cook knows, a judicious blend of contrasting tastes can help turn otherwise bland dietary staples into great tasting food. Often, the same interplay between sweet and sour that energizes wine is part of the magic behind savory dishes that also stimulate our appetites with warm seasonings and piquant flavors. Savory tastes are particularly evident in Asian cuisines, which tend to rely less on heavy preparations with large pieces of meat and more on lighter vegetables and broths. Popular dishes in many other cuisines also employ an artful tension between sweet and sour to bring some excitement to the dish, such as chocolate, marmalade or cranberry sauce. To some extent, the basic principle applies to just about every combination beyond meat and potatoes.

For dishes that involve a contrast between sweet and sour, you can employ an approach similar to that used in matching body and texture. It's obvious that sweet on sweet will suffocate, and bitter on bitter will disrupt, the other flavors in your meal. Where the sweet taste is the dominant one, the wine will need to have enough acidity to hold its own. For dishes where sour dominates, you'll need a sweeter wine so you're not overcome by the sourness of the dish. Where the food is more balanced itself, you will want to use a balanced wine and concentrate on the marriage of flavor elements just the way the winemaker does with the wine. Asian cuisines often rely on both bold, contrasting flavors and subtle, earthy ones. New-world-style wines, including intensely flavored reds like Pinot Noir, tend to work best where the bold contrasts dominate, while an earthier dish will often pair better with spicier, old-world-style whites, such as Gewürztraminers, and dry, herbaceous rosés.

The Acid Test

Earlier, I've shown you how acidity plays a major role in determining a wine's structure, texture and flavor. As you become more proficient at matching, you'll notice that underlying acidity is often the key that unlocks the most satisfying pairings. Just the right touch of acidity stimulates the taste buds and helps bring out the flavor in many dishes, particularly those that have delicate flavors. But a wine that's too high in acid can put a metallic edge on dishes that include foods like liver or kidneys and can otherwise distract from the sweet unctuousness of other dark meats. So the ability to judge the level of acidity in a wine is useful for good food and wine pairing.

Judging overall acidity can be a bit tricky, however. As we've seen, there are different kinds of acids in wine, which play different roles in contributing to its structure, texture and flavor. Remember that the impact of citric, malic and tannic acids on a wine changes over time and that the word "acidity" is used in different ways. As a general characteristic, acidity almost always refers to the basic sour acidity that comes from tartaric acid, while for food and wine matching it's the "total acidity" at the time it's being consumed that's most important to you.

If a wine is young, its brighter acids and tannins won't have broken down as much and they'll add significantly to total acidity. As wine ages, however, its tannins and other acids break down. The total acidity will abate and the sourness of the more durable tartaric acid in the wine will tend to dominate its taste. This is why fruity, late maturing varieties like Cabernet Sauvignon, Syrah and Tempranillo are ideal components of a wine that's made to age, and also why having the best sites and good harvests is so important for making age-worthy wines from varieties like Pinot Noir, Nebbiolo and Sangiovese, whose natural acidity makes them a good match for foods in general, but whose affinity for cool climates sometimes means that they don't ripen fully before they are picked.

There is acidity in many foods, and the wines we drink with them need to maintain a corresponding level of acidity in order not to feel flaccid by comparison. Acidity in food typically comes from fruit (including foods like tomatoes and peppers that are not usually thought of as fruits) and dairy products (including baked goods made with milk and butter, as well as cheeses, yogurt, buttermilk and custards). When matching foods that are lower in acidity, it's usually a good idea to use a lower-acid wine, or the food will taste less exciting.

It's also important to distinguish tannic acidity from dryness when matching wines with sweeter foods. An extremely dry wine can provide too much of a contrast and clash with a sweet dish, while a wine that's too sweet can seem cloying. But remember the special impact that tannic acid has on the texture of a wine. It's important not to confuse the rough, dry feeling that tannins leave in your mouth with true dryness in a wine, which is the absence of residual sugar that occurs when most of the sugar in the grapes has been converted into alcohol by fermentation. The amount of residual sugar in a wine isn't always apparent in a tannic wine, because a significant amount of sweetness can lie hidden under the tannins. Just because it feels drying to the tongue doesn't mean that a wine will contrast well with sweeter foods.

Why Wine Critics Prefer Low-Acid Wines

It's particularly useful to keep acidity in mind when you drink wine without food, because that little extra touch of acid that makes a wine food-friendly can seem a bit harsh all by itself. In head-to-head comparisons without food, wines with lower acidity will often taste better. Typically, we pay the most attention to a wine when we first drink it and that is often before we eat any food. Those critical first impressions can be a bit misleading if we're trying to judge whether the wine is suitable for a meal and forget to concentrate on the amount of acidity that might be needed to stand up to the dishes we'll be consuming with it later.

Wine critics typically prefer to taste wine without much more distraction than a crust of bread. It's understandable that someone with a good palate would resist being "trained" or "educated" to prefer higher-acid wines when it doesn't come naturally. Their readers are also most likely to evaluate their recommendations when taking their first sip of a wine before a meal or when a retailer offers a sample in the wine shop. Here the match is environmental—consumer and critic taste the wine under similar circumstances, i.e., without food.

Because lower-acid wines are generally more pleasing in a controlled tasting environment, it's understandable that many consumers are confused by the disconnect between what they hear from critics about various wines and what they experience when they try to match them with foods. Like me, they may also find that their favorite wines seem less pleasing when they taste them with food and blame the mismatch on food's general unfriendliness to wine, rather than on a mismatch between the lower acidity in the wine and the higher acidity in the food they're tasting with it. When sampling wines at the point of sale or choosing them on the basis of a critic's review, remember that your impressions may not be a reliable guide to their ability to pair with a meal due to the absence of food at the tasting.

The End Game: Finer Match Points

Among the most important qualities of a grape variety from the perspective of food pairing is its ability to mimic the tastes of various fruits, herbs, nuts and spices. As you become familiar with varietal flavors in various wines, you'll see many opportunities to use these to blend with and accent the flavors in your food. In this respect, wine can serve as a liquid condiment and can play the same sort of role in a meal that spices, sauces and side dishes do. A wine that tastes lemony will do well with a fish you squeeze lemons on, while a meat dish typically served with a mint sauce will do well with a wine that leaves a slightly minty taste in your mouth.

As you develop your food and wine pairing skills, pay particular attention to how different grape varietals recreate the impression of various foods. Here again comparison tasting with everyday foods and wines will be useful as you begin to master the fine points, since you'll be able to apply what you learn more often and build on it. One unusual but surprisingly effective way to learn about pairings is to put together a selection of foods from a local fast food outlet. These outlets usually specialize in preparing the same basic food, such as chicken, fish or beef (or in the case of pizza, bread), in several different ways, such as with and without cheese, or with different sauces and condiments. This can provide an inexpensive way to see how different preparations of a single food affect its ability to pair with different varietals. People are usually surprised by how much difference the type of preparation makes to a food and wine pairing and may find a new appreciation for some varietals that they haven't had much experience with before as a result of this exercise.

If you have an inclination to try this, keep in mind that you'll be ordering more food and wine than you need, so you may want to invite some adventuresome friends along. If your friends have the time and inclination to do a bit of work, you can also do this exercise with more nutritious and delicious food. Pick a food that can be prepared in various different ways and assign each of your friends a different dish and a different type of wine. Then mix and match. Either way you arrange it, there are likely to be some lively interactions you can learn from.

You can also gain insights into pairings by becoming more familiar with the relationships between regional cuisines and the wines that are identified with the region. Many regional cuisines have been developed in tandem with regional wines. This has given rise to another helpful slogan (again a reminder, not a rule): "What grows together, goes together." You can use an understanding of that to match wines from a particular region with the traditional dishes of the region and use what you observe to add to your bag of pairing tricks. In this regard, it's also useful to develop a somewhat more nuanced view of the differences between old-world and new-world preferences. Within the different European and new-world wine regions, there are differences in emphasis from one region to another. Where the French prefer dry wines and emphasize earthy qualities, Germans tolerate more sweetness and emphasize minerality, while Italian wines tend to be more bitter and Spanish wines fruitier.

These preferences are often reflected in new-world wine styles as well. Argentinean, Chilean and Californian producers generally make fruitier wines, perhaps because of residual influences from the Spanish missionaries who first planted grapes in these regions (although the Argentines have also been influenced by Italian immigration). Australians and New Zealanders have been influenced not only by the English love of beer, but also their broad appreciation of wines from all of Europe's wine-producing countries. Perhaps the absence of a typically British wine style is responsible for the more eclectic and scientifically oriented approach to viticulture and winemaking in Australia and New Zealand. The South Africans, on the other hand, were heavily influenced by the Dutch. The Dutch didn't make their own wine, but had a long been involved in the wine trade in the Loire Valley and Bordeaux and brought winemakers from these areas to South Africa.

Taking it to the Next Level

I've listed a number of food and wine pairings in Appendix C. The first group of pairings is intended to help you identify the varietals that you might want to concentrate on. By locating the foods you enjoy and seeing which varietals show up most often, you may be able to get a sense of which varietals are most likely to appeal to your palate. Because it lists only varietals and not specific wines, and identifies foods rather than prepared dishes, this list will be of use only as a starting point for understanding food and wine pairings.

To give you a sense of how glorious food and wine pairings can ultimately be, I've also provided a short list of some classic food and wine pairings. This second listing is more specific about the wines and the dishes in the match. It's a straightforward listing without much commentary. I can't tell you *exactly* why these pairings work because I'm sure I don't really know. I wouldn't be surprised or even disappointed to find that *no one* really knows. That's what makes them special.

It would be surprising if these combinations don't work for you, however, even though they'll work for you in a way that is different from everyone else. Trying them, and trying to figure out the reasons they appeal to you and so many others, should be a useful way to develop your understanding of pairings. Be careful to remember, however, that all the suggestions in Appendix C necessarily reflect the idiosyncrasies of my palate. Don't expect to experience them exactly the way I do.

Stay Systematic

As you branch out in your experiments with wine and food, blind luck will turn up a fair number of surprisingly good matches. Unfortunately, as you get more adventuresome, the odds of a mismatch can also increase. To decrease the chances of that, develop an approach that lets you experiment in a systematic way. If you're with others, try to remember that the most important task is to match the occasion. Don't stretch for an exotic combination just to see what it's like unless the others you're with are in the mood for that as well. When you have the opportunity to drink a great wine, play it safe and stick to the classic foods that are known to go well with it. You don't want to ruin everyone else's meal or your enjoyment of a rare wine just to teach yourself a lesson.

While you're taking care of others, others will be taking care of you. Most good restaurants will make sure the wines they offer, particularly those by the glass, complement the signature flavors of the foods they serve. After all, since wine can greatly enhance the customer's appreciation of the food, it's natural to try to increase the odds of a good selection by the customers. One of the main reasons most folks never get beyond the old "white with fish, red with meat" rule is probably because, when they use it in a restaurant, it works pretty well most of the time.

Just as you became adept at knowing what to expect from various wines simply by noticing how they taste, you can easily develop a knack for better food and wine pairings simply by paying attention to the interactions between the wines you drink and the foods you eat. Remember that food and wine pairing isn't only about those perfect combinations that food and wine writers swoon over; it's mostly about making the best match you can out of what you have available. Concentrate on the short game and you'll be impressed with rapid the improvement in your score.

Use What You've Learned

You may not appreciate it yet, but in the course of reading this book you've already acquired most of the basic skills needed to make better pairings of food and wine. The most fundamental one is the ability to appreciate the flavor and feel of the wines you drink. The *sine qua non* of conscious pairing, as compared with blind luck, is being able to anticipate the taste of a wine so you can imagine how it might match with a particular food. Then it's a fairly straightforward process to compare the choices you have available and zero in on the ones with the best chance to work.

With so many foods and ways to prepare them, as well as so many different wines, proper matching can seem a bit intimidating. All that diversity makes for thousands of pairings, some great and some awful, and focusing on them one by one will only lead you on a long and merry chase. Just as with wines themselves, focusing on a few exotic pairings won't help much with your everyday needs. Knowing that a late-harvest Romorantin can make a startlingly good combination with *washugyu* is interesting and may earn you points with your oenophile friends, but most of us can't find or afford either of them very often.

It's better to think of that kind of pairing as pleasant entertainment. To enhance your ordinary food and wine pairings, concentrate on how to handle the fussy foods, match body and texture and avoid clashes between the dominant players. These are skills you can use every day and they'll still be useful if you decide to make wine and food matching into your favorite sport.

The Sublime and the Ordinary

As you experiment with wine pairings for the foods you eat most often, you'll find some that will become personal favorites. Occasionally, you'll also stumble across spectacular pairings for foods you don't eat every day. These needn't be exotic foods. Some of the best pairings involve relatively tasteless foods that suddenly come alive when combined with the right wine.

Experiencing just one perfect pairing can start you off on a lifetime of pleasurable experimentation, seeking to recapture the thrill again and again. You've nothing to lose, and your meals will just get better and better. But you don't need to spend years in search of food and wine nirvana to enjoy the benefits of everyday food-and-wine matching. If you keep the basics in mind, it won't take you long to learn how to make successful matches even when you have limited choices available.

People feel they know the foods they like and how they'll taste, but many find wines a bit of a challenge. In one frequently mentioned study, researchers at the University of California (Davis) tested a group of ordinary consumers by putting red and white wines in black mugs and found that few could tell the difference between the wines. Now that you're near the end of this book, however, you needn't labor under this handicap.

Whether you can see the color of a wine or not, you can pay attention to its aromas, flavors and textures. As you become familiar with a broader range of wines, your pairing palette will become more diverse and you'll learn when to use a broad stroke or just a touch of accent. With experience, you'll begin to develop a sixth sense for the pairings that work best for you and, like me, you'll start to wonder why so many others never develop it.

Like any creative instinct, the instinct for pairing is sharpened by both trusting and protecting it. It's fairly easy to learn how to scan the menu for fussy foods and concentrate on the textures and dominant notes in food and wine. Developing these routines will eliminate most of the nasty surprises that erode your confidence. As your confidence builds, it will be increasingly natural to trust your instincts and you'll be increasingly reminded that good pairings aren't simply a matter of matching wines to foods. They're a way to exploit the best a wine has to offer, so you can enhance special occasions and make ordinary occasions special. Keep your attention on the people you're sharing your wine with. Think about where you are and the mood you want to sustain. Remember to match these with care and your wine will be as good as it gets.

Not Talking About It

To receive, get open

Wine is one of the most discussed topics in history. Homer spoke of "wild wine" that makes "the wisest man sing at the top of his lungs" and tempts him to "blurt out stories better never told." Ever since, the subject of wine has found a prominent place in Western literature. Today, any bookstore is likely to have a small collection of wine books for everyone from the beginner to the fanatic. There is a thriving wine media, including a small army of bloggers who probe the intimate details of each wine region, harvest and producer. Winemakers and sommeliers have become celebrities in their own right.

So with all that attention to wine, how can I say that people don't talk about it enough?

Here's the problem: only a few people are doing most of the talking, and it's not the ones who really need to do it the most. When we're reading a book or magazine, we aren't in a situation where we really *need* to talk about wine. We might enjoy reading about it and sharing what we learn with someone else, but we don't really *need* to talk about it then and there.

When we do need to talk about wine is when we're in the process of choosing it. That's when we have to sort through all the different factors involved and can get hung up on one or another of them. Sharing a few thoughts with someone else can help put things into a better perspective.

Just at this point, however, too many people observe an awkward silence. The clerk in the shop asks, "Are you looking for anything special today?" With a shake of the head and a friendly wave, the customer quietly shuffles toward the other end of the store (where a shrewd retailer will put the most expensive wines). The waiter asks, "Would you like me to send the sommelier over?" and the diner defers, perhaps not realizing that the expense of the sommelier's services is built into the cost of the wine, whether they're used or not.

There are a number of reasons why people get tongue-tied about wine at the moment of choice, but the main one seems to be fear of embarrassment. Wine seems a lot like sex: you hear so much hype, it's hard to find the right words for a little honest talk.

The Silent Selector

Here's a situation that you've probably observed fairly often. A couple or a group enters a restaurant and is seated. Soon the server appears with menus and asks about the wine list. Everyone defers to the host or someone else who's supposed to know more about wine than they do. When asked if any help would be useful in choosing a wine, this person declines, quietly reading the wine list and making a selection without any discussion with anyone else at the table.

There may be occasions when this is appropriate. The group might be too large or the restaurant too noisy to solicit input from others profitably. More often, however, it's a sign that the person choosing the wine doesn't know much more about it than anyone else.

It's particularly amusing to see this play out with certain traditional couples. The silent selector usually ends up paying the bill, but it's the person on the other side of the table who knows about food and how it's prepared. Even if our silent selector does know more about wine, isn't worthwhile to get some insights from across the table about the food?

Even worse, whether it's a couple or a larger group, it's quite common that our silent selector will make the choice of wine without knowing what anyone will be eating. This is not only inconsiderate to the others but a clue that the silent selector is clueless. How can someone have any idea what a wine will taste like and not be aware of how that taste can be changed by what they and others might eat?

Signals for Silence

The silent selection of wine is tolerated to an extent that suggests that there is more than politeness at work. Many professionals in the wine trade blame the customer for not responding to their offers of assistance, but they fail to realize the subtle signals they themselves give to reinforce this behavior.

For example, restaurants will often ask if the wine has been chosen before anyone has had a chance to review the menu. If the group is there to drink wine without regard to the food they're eating, they'd be better off in a wine bar. And if they don't think the wine has anything to do with how they enjoy their meal, they should probably order something else. Asking for the wine order before the food is selected necessarily implies that the wine is merely a detail to be attended to quickly before the main event gets underway.

Restaurants enable silent selections in other ways as well. People can't be blamed for deferring to someone else when the server brings only one wine list to the table, especially if there are no wines listed on the menu. The list is difficult to pass around. Handing out just one is an implicit suggestion that specialization is in order; that most people are presumed to know what they like in food, but need help when it comes to the wine.

Although it was fairly common just ten years ago for a restaurant server to simply hand the wine list to the oldest male at the table, this happens much less frequently today. (If it does, other aspects of their service may be a bit antiquated too.) More frequently, the server will ask who should receive the wine list or will discreetly place it somewhere on the table where it's reasonably accessible to anyone. Sometimes a few wines from the list that might pair well with the specials will actually be listed next to them on the menus that everyone receives. At some really enlightened establishments, everyone gets the list, which makes sense to me. How likely is it that they would give only one person a menu? They don't share menus even in restaurants where people are expected to share food.

By handing out only a single wine list, restaurants actively discourage people from talking about their wine. Some go further by not having anyone available to discuss the wines intelligently with the customers. For the most part, these restaurants would be better off just getting rid of their list...and their wines. Why an establishment with a good list should want to discourage customers from talking about it is a mystery to me.

Mixed Messages

There are other situations where curious omissions in what is said about wine can create confusion for reasons that might be a bit easier to understand. These are events at which there's quite a bit of talk about wine, but little or none about its taste. Ironically, these are often called wine tastings and may be sponsored by wine publications, wine societies, chefs or retailers. The theme may be the wines of a particular illustrious region or producer. The wines are always good to excellent and are usually presented with a meal or snack specifically chosen to match the wines. Often the meal itself is worth more than the price of admission. I enjoy these events, because many of the people who attend are enthusiastic about wine and like talking about it.

The focus at these events is certainly on the wines, but for a variety of reasons the conversation dances around the ultimate question of their taste. They often feature speakers who represent the producer or producers whose wines are featured. These speakers are generally very knowledgeable about the wines. Unfortunately, however, the focus of their remarks is rarely on the taste of the wine or how it pairs with the food (which is usually treated as something of a state secret). What the audience usually hears about is trivia, interesting for the wine connoisseur, but confusing and not very helpful for the ordinary consumer.

The speakers at these events typically confine their remarks to the history of the vineyards and the family or company making the wines, focusing particularly on legendary personalities from the past or trendsetting celebrities in the present. Perhaps the region that the wines are from will be discussed, including the topography, climate and characteristic grape varieties. The unique qualities of the weather during certain vintages may also be discussed. These are all things the astute consumers in the audience should find interesting, but they should also be interested in the taste of the wines, which is rarely mentioned.

One could argue that it's reasonable not to talk about the taste of the wines, since everyone's tastes are different. But any serious wine drinker is interested in what wines taste like and doesn't mind hearing someone else's opinion about it. The reason taste isn't mentioned isn't because the members of the audience aren't interested in it or want to make up their own mind. In fact, it may be precisely because they are interested and might not hesitate to disagree with the speaker that the speaker avoids the subject.

Talking about the taste of the wines at these events might open the door for someone to say something that might be controversial or upsetting to the principal speaker or sponsor of the event. It's also not the time to mention what the critic who gave high marks to the wine actually wrote about the taste, because the participants might be disappointed that they don't actually seem to taste as good as they sound. But between these fears and the fear that discussing the food pairings will somehow dim the luster of the wines, one can easily be left with the wrong impression. You might think that knowing the history of the producer, the vagaries of the vintages and the idiosyncrasies of the personalities involved are more important than knowing what the wine tastes like.

Wine tastings are often assumed to be opportunities for people to become educated about wine. Unfortunately, it takes a fairly well-educated consumer to make good use of the information provided at these events. Whether the event is a massive charity event with dozens of lesser-quality wines or an intimate dinner with the winemaker for a prestigious domain, it's likely that many people who attend will actually leave more confused than better educated.

If you do take advantage of these events, and you should, there is no reason why you shouldn't make note of the taste of the wines. Usually, a private moment will present itself where you can talk to the sponsor or a featured speaker about your impressions. They are usually quite happy to discuss the matter with you offline. You can learn a great deal and no one's feathers will be ruffled.

Old Biases—New Hype

From Roman times, the control that the European aristocracy has exercised over the land, and thus the favored plots for growing grapes, has created an association between the nobility of the vineyard owner and the quality of their wines. Their ownership of castles and grand estates, with cool cellars for storing the wines, has inevitably reinforced the association. As a result, many European producers, and the new-world producers who emulate them, make an effort to promote their wines by emphasizing their connection to nobility.

This connection may be real or imaginary, but in either case it has little to do with taste or quality in the world of wine today. Sometimes the effort can be a bit comical, too, as when the owner of a lesser château boasts to a wine journalist that its wine makes a perfect match for braised geese-hearts or some other obscure hunter's dish. That this type of imagery continues to have such a visible place in wine lore and marketing is bound to give additional mixed signals to the average wine drinker. In particular, it creates a public image of wine producers and wine lovers as disconnected from reality and of the rituals of wine merely as vestiges of an earlier age.

To a novice, the rituals of wine often can also seem either daunting or silly and a bit exclusionary. However, most people who understand the rituals of wine love to share them because they serve useful purposes. They are ways of facilitating the enjoyment of wine and creating bonds among those who love it. They can also facilitate the interactions between consumers and producers, allow them to understand each other better and let them share their mutual appreciation of nature's bounty and their respective roles in nurturing it.

The disciples of wine cling to its traditions the way a bishop clings to a crosier, as a symbol of their connection to the great family of past, present and future wine lovers and their pastoral concern for the vineyards and the people who support them. Useful as they may be, however, the traditions of the wine world can be somewhat removed from what we need to know to enjoy wine better. Treating them as mystical secrets passed down among the cognoscenti can leave a newcomer to wine scratching his or her head in bewilderment or, worse, thinking that there really isn't a wizard behind the curtain.

Learning to Understand Winespeak

Another thing that confuses and intimidates people about wine is the specialized vocabulary that professionals use to describe it. As with any other area of endeavor, the world of wine has its own culture and vocabulary and wine writing has certain conventions that anyone who wants to reach a wine-loving audience finds it useful to adopt. Just as it takes a while to learn the rules and the jargon before you can enjoy watching a sporting event or follow the play action commentary of it in the media, it takes a while to absorb the traditions and talk of the wine trade.

Once they understand them, most people find the vocabulary and conventions used by wine writers useful, take pride in their knowledge and enjoy the feeling of being among the select few who are in the know. But that can make others feel a bit left out.

If you're familiar with the typical tasting notes written by wine reviewers and columnists, you may have noticed that the descriptions in this book are somewhat different. Although I've stressed the importance of being able to taste wine, I haven't described the taste of specific wines by reference to the specific fruits, vegetables and spices. Instead, I've mentioned broad *categories* like citrus, spice, "red fruits" and "dark fruits." The reason for this is that I haven't assumed that you're familiar with the vocabulary and conventions of the wine media.

Since everyone's palate is different, a lemon or a blackberry will taste different to you than it does to a wine reviewer, particularly if you haven't become familiar with the way descriptions of various fruits, vegetables, herbs and spices serve as code words for flavors and other tastes in wine that are similar. It's also quite likely that one wine will taste somewhat, or even significantly, different from another, even if it's made from the same grapes, in the same region, at the same time. Indeed, there is often "bottle variation," differences between bottles of wine with identical labels, caused by the fact that the producer did not blend all the wines from various casks or batches together before bottling or by differences in the way the wines were handled and stored after bottling.

So it's a real challenge for wine writers to describe the taste of a wine in a way that the everyday consumer will relate to. To make it easier, they rely on a consensus that has been worked out over the centuries about how to describe the tastes that are characteristic in various wines. If you want to understand them, it helps to have an idea about what that consensus is about.

When we discussed varietal flavors, I explained that the descriptions of flavors in wine are only approximations. When a wine writer, retailer, sommelier, or serious wine devotee refers to a wine as tasting like cherries, they don't expect you to believe that the wine tastes exactly like cherries. Rather, they're saying that the wine has a taste in it that makes most serious wine drinkers think of cherries. It takes not only time and practice to be able to pick that taste out, but also some familiarity with the consensus view of what that taste is in a wine.

When you first discover the flavor element in wine that others refer to as cherries, it might seem only vaguely related to what cherries taste like to you. After making the association several times, however, you'll feel more and more comfortable thinking of it as a cherry taste. In the case of most fruits, the taste that experts refer to is more subtle and dried than the taste we experience when we eat the fruit fresh. So, what wine professionals refer to as "educating the palate" is not a process of training the taste buds and olfactory nerves to work more efficiently. Rather it's a process of learning the conventions wine professionals use when they refer to a particular taste in a wine.

Wine reviewers also use a variety of tricks to tease tastes out of a wine that are not in the forefront when you drink it normally. They will swirl it, sniff it deeply up into the epithelium and roll it around on their tongue while they suck in air and chew on it, making a scene that you wouldn't want to make at the dinner table. They will also let the wine warm up beyond the normal serving temperature, because that's where its virtues and flaws will both be more evident. All of these things allow a professional to identify tastes in the wine that may seem quite faint to the average wine drinker, or be experienced only subliminally.

It's not surprising then that many people ignore what wine writers say about the taste of the wine. To make things even more confusing, many wine writers and other wine professionals work to distinguish themselves by developing ever more impressive and complex descriptions, making it hard for the average consumer to even figure out the consensus view. The rapport that great writers have with their readers can make their descriptions become part of the consensus view. But they also have many eager imitators. These imitators may someday become great wine critics in their own right, but in the meantime, they can simply add to the confusion by trying a bit too hard to get your attention.

You'll find it easier to understand wine writing if you keep in mind that all descriptions of wine are an offering to the collective consciousness of wine tasters. Treat them as if you were tasting wine with some friends and sharing opinions. The views of professionals might be better researched and better expressed (they have to be, since they can't talk back when you disagree). But they shouldn't be treated as guarantees of what a wine should taste like to you. Think of them merely as suggestions based on experience. Try to connect these views with the tastes that you find in your wines, but don't expect to taste exactly what you first expect when you hear the description. It may take a while for you to see what a professional is talking about. It's also possible that it's just not there when you taste the wine or that you just can't taste it for some reason. That shouldn't prevent you from thinking about what you do taste.

You don't need to sound like a wine writer to talk to friends and family about wine, and you shouldn't need to use winespeak to talk to a wine professional either. Wary of the oversimplifications that jargon lends itself to, most true wine professionals will only use winespeak when it helps to simplify things or as a shorthand to make communications with other professionals more efficient. They are much more interested in discussing things that are out of the ordinary about a wine, rather than the predictable consensus view. These are the kind of fresh perspectives that winespeak hasn't assimilated yet, so it doesn't hurt to talk about what you taste in your own words even when you're discussing wine with a pro.

Making Sense of Wine Reviews

Bear in mind that there should be a difference between written and oral winespeak. Written winespeak, like good dialog, only simulates natural talk. Its main value lies in how it serves to carry the underlying message to the audience. Yet the different audiences that written winespeak is addressed to sometimes require it to be unduly complicated. Take for example the typical tasting note. Here's one from the October 2010 issue of the *Wine Spectator* for the 2007 Opus One:

> Tight and firm, with a chewy edge to the dried currant, graphite, blackberry and mineral notes. Full-bodied and intense, without being weighty, this is well-structured with a complex, persistent finish. Cabernet Sauvignon, Merlot, Cabernet Franc, Petit Verdot and Malbec...94

This is a review that says everything and not very much. It's a concise and accurate description of the wine directed principally to the broad audience of people who will read it in displays on retailers' shelves or in their advertising materials. That's an audience that may or may not know much about wine. Nevertheless, it's an important audience for the *Wine Spectator*, as it is for other critics, since retailers pay a fee to use these tasting notes in their advertisements. Because that audience is so broad, the note has to include information that seems obvious to many wine drinkers (and presumably most of the *Wine Spectator*'s actual subscribers).

If you glanced at Appendix B when you were reading the previous chapter, you may have noticed that flavors of *currants, blackberries* and *graphite* are typical of wines made from the grape varieties listed in this review. Blending them will make the wine more *complex,* and a *persistent finish* is characteristic of wines made from Cabernet Sauvignon, the variety that's listed first and the first you would expect to find in a wine made in Napa Valley, California. You would also expect these wines to spend some time in oak barrels, enhancing the sense of *graphite* (which we associate with cedar pencil shavings) and bringing out the *dry* tannins in the wines, which might be described as making it seem *tighter* and *firmer* and, without too much poetic license, even *"chewy."*

Since this wine is made by a consortium started by leading producers from the Napa Valley and Bordeaux, one would expect them to have produced a *well-structured* wine, which means, as the review says, that it fills the mouth (*full-bodied*) without leaving it overwhelmed (*being weighty*). Since 2007 was an extremely good year in Napa Valley, the flavors in the wines can be expected to be *intense.*

Did I leave anything out? Go back and check. What this review in the *Wine Spectator* is saying is simply that the wine is what it should be.

Because there is a bias toward writing wine reviews that will be informative to less knowledgeable consumers, most informed consumers pay more attention to what wine reviews don't say than what they do say. Here, the review doesn't mention the color of the wine or any overtones of pepper or spiciness. That's interesting because one of the grape varieties used here, Petit Verdot, is known for bringing these qualities to the wine. It's also difficult to grow and customarily associated more with wines from the Médoc in France than with wines from Napa Valley.

A knowledgeable wine consumer might ask whether the effort that has been made to include Petit Verdot in this wine has been worth it. But let's not judge based on just one review. Let's look at what the legendary Robert Parker has to say. After all, he made his early reputation based primarily on his knowledge of wines from the Médoc and is also credited with being a major force in popularizing the wines of Napa Valley around the world. Here is a review of the same wine that Parker wrote when he tasted in December of 2008:

> A wine that may approach the prototypically perfect idea of what Opus One wants to be is the 2007. Production was down by at least 20%, and the result is a wine with extraordinary concentration of crème de cas-

sis intermixed with licorice, cedarwood, and spice box. It reveals dazzling purity of fruit on the attack and mid-palate, builds to a full-bodied, sumptuous mouthfeel, and closes with a long, 50+ second finish. This 2007 has the potential to be the finest Opus One ever made since the first vintage in 1979…94-97

One thing that you'll notice here is that Parker's prose is rather evocative in comparison to the more straightforward approach of the previous review. Crème de cassis sounds a bit more exotic than dried currants, although he's describing the same taste. He picks up on the cedar, rather than the graphite, which sounds a bit more appetizing as well. Adjectives like *prototypically perfect, dazzling* and *sumptuous* don't add much to our understanding of the wine, but they do help to convey some of his enthusiasm for the wine and make me, at least, wish I had a glass in hand, right now!

Parker's review also conveys a sense of rigor and detail. He provides an explanation for why the 2007 wines from Napa are extraordinary (the weather conditions produced tighter, firmer grapes with 20 percent less juice) and the finish has been timed almost down to the second. These details help us decide for ourselves what he means by his descriptions.

Parker's knack for detailed yet evocative prose is undoubt-edly what has earned him legions of fans and the gratitude of countless producers, importers and retailers, if not the entire nation of France. But does his review convey more than the fact that the wine is as it should be?

In that respect, Parker's review is not significantly different from the one in the *Wine Spectator*. He does mention the "spice box" that he often also finds in wines from the Médoc that include Petit Verdot in the blend. It's a useful addition, if you're wondering about the Petit Verdot question, but not entirely unexpected.

What these reviews exemplify, and Parker's particularly, is the simple fact that, if you have to state the obvious, you might as well do it in an entertaining way. This is symptomatic of a much broader bias toward the positive in wine writing, for which there are various reasons.

Bias in the Grape Press

Despite their legendary ability to pick up a touch of truffle in the taste or hint of violets in the aroma, I've never read a wine review that detected the flavor of grape juice concentrate, beet sugar or any of the other additives sometimes used in making wine. Yet these additions are not that uncommon and are used by many reputable producers to round out the taste or correct a minor flaw in a wine. This is true even in areas such as Europe, where there is a general bias against wines that are "manipulated."

Reviews also rarely talk about other common flaws, such as those discussed in Appendix A. They're not, as you'll see, unknown, even among more expensive wines, yet they're rarely mentioned in reviews. One assumes that they are either treated as one-off experiences when they happen or that the wines the reviewers taste have been carefully screened not to include them.

Undoubtedly, a natural bias against discussing embarrassing details is also engendered by the inevitable personal relationships that are formed between wine writers and wine producers. In addition, given the prominence of Europeans in the ranks of both producers and writers, one might expect a certain cultural bias toward avoiding the unpleasant. The blunt musings of a critic might be seen as simply part of the job in the United States. In France or Italy, however, where people are expected to be more polite in their formal exchanges, those same musings might spark a lawsuit, and the producer could win it.

Cronyism and cultural differences may play a part, but it seems obvious that the main reason for wine writing to be skewed to the positive is that readers are used to it that way. Since most wine writing is intended for readers who are wine lovers and supported by advertisers who are producers or distributors, it isn't surprising that wine writing has a positive bias or that readers will get used to it being that way. I've lost track of the number of people who've told me not to include the next chapter because readers will want an introductory wine book to be unremittingly positive.

When you combine the razzle-dazzle it takes for a wine writer to get noticed with an industry-wide bias toward saying positive things about wine, its easy to see why you don't need, and in fact shouldn't try, to sound like a wine critic. You certainly don't want to spend eighty percent of your time figuring out creative ways to state the obvious over and over and make it sound new and exciting. But most of all, you do want to talk about the bad stuff, because that could easily interfere with your enjoyment of a wine you're about to select. To make the best choices, you'll also need to talk a bit about yourself, which always seems pretentious in the media.

Starting the Conversation

There's another imposing barrier you might need to overcome before you feel comfortable about speaking up when you're choosing a wine. In addition to worrying about your lack of knowledge or familiarity with winespeak, you'll often be talking to a complete stranger. It's always hard to talk to a stranger, especially when you have to reveal something about yourself and may have reason to fear that this stranger might not have your best interests at heart.

Let me reassure you a bit. While your fear of their self-interest isn't entirely irrational, there are many reasons why shopkeepers and sommeliers who don't know you have as much interest in selling you wines that provide good value as those with a high profit margin.

The first, of course, is that at the outset of the conversation they know as little about you as you know about them. So it's safer for them to begin with the assumption that you're a knowledgeable consumer. After all, if they assume the reverse and are wrong, it won't exactly start things off on a good footing.

Remember that every time you select a wine there is a match to be made and that your own needs and preferences will be the most important determinant of what works best for you. So just saying a bit about what you need is a good way to get the conversation started. That doesn't say anything about a particular wine, but it's a signal that you have your priorities straight.

You'll find a curious difference between what you actually say and what they hear. For example, you might be with a party of four in a restaurant. If you simply acknowledge the difficulty of choosing a wine to complement all the different dishes being ordered, it will be interpreted as a mark of discernment. The server knows he or she should have a deeper understanding of all of those dishes than you do and should rise to the occasion. The presumption will be made that you're knowledgeable about wine even though you haven't said anything about it.

If the restaurant is in a wine region or features the food of a particular region, you could comment quite honestly about how you're looking forward to learning more about the wines of that region. The server will tend to hear something that suggests that you know a fair amount about wine, but just haven't had the opportunity to try the wines from this region before. In fact, after reading this book, you probably know more about wines than you think and the conversation will proceed quite amicably. You now know there are no absolute rules about wine. As long as you keep things simple, you're unlikely to give away any lack of knowledge on your part.

Once you do get the conversation started, however, it's relatively easy to learn enough about clerks in a shop or wine servers in the restaurants to know whether you'll benefit from taking their advice. Just see whether the advice makes sense because they're talking about the taste of the wine and asking about what you like, rather than talking about who the producer is, what a good deal the wine is or how much other customers have liked it. If they veer off into unfamiliar territory in the course of the discussion, bring them back into your own frame of reference by mentioning a wine you've had recently, no matter how modest or obscure it might be. Real professionals want to hear about the wines you drink, because it's a way to get to know you on terms they can relate to best. They're even likely to see some connection between that and whatever they were just talking about, even if it seems to be a rather abrupt turn in the conversation to you.

Nine times out of ten, when someone projects a superior attitude about their knowledge of wine, it's intended to intimidate you and cover up their own lack of knowledge. You can safely take whatever they say with a large grain of salt. Likewise, if they give you a hard sell, it's because they want to make the sale before you realize what might be wrong. But snobbishness and hard sells are rare exceptions in my experience. If they don't act superior or pushy, there's good reason to listen to what retailers and restaurateurs have to say about wine. You're more likely to visit them again if you've found their advice helpful.

The Price Point

It's always good to share some information about the price you're prepared to pay when you're buying a wine. You can usually do this in a way that gets the seller on your side. You might say: "Usually, we can't really afford to drink the better wines from the XYZ region, but since we love these wines and are celebrating a special occasion, we thought perhaps today we could afford to stretch things a tiny bit." Since most of the people who serve you also love wine and are on a limited budget themselves, you'll establish an immediate bond that will work to your advantage.

If you're offered a taste of wine in a shop or restaurant, accepting it is a great way to start the conversation about what you like. If it's being offered to you, it's a safe bet that it's also being offered to others and it's unlikely to be a high-priced wine. So you needn't feel shy about accepting a taste without buying it. Your reaction to the taste can be a useful reference point in your discussions, even if the wine turns out to be above the price point you are looking for at that particular time. If the taste of the wine appeals to you, you can say so, and ask how it might or might not fit in with what you're looking for. If the response makes sense, you may have found a new wine to enjoy. If it doesn't, you can feel comfortable that you won't miss out on anything by choosing a different wine on your own. Meanwhile, thinking a bit about why that wine is being recommended could give you valuable information about the wine and the caliber of the establishment.

It may be that you don't like a wine that you've been given to taste. Don't be afraid to say so and give the reason. You could simply take a sip and say immediately that the wine isn't to your taste, but that's likely to end the conversation. Before you comment, make a point of showing that you're looking at the wine. Then swirl it around, let it warm up a bit and give it a good sniff before tasting it slowly. It's both a courtesy and a sign of discernment to take your time when you're offered a taste of wine.

During the time you're swirling and nosing the wine, you can think up a question, even something as innocuous as "Have you been getting a good response to this?" Any open-ended question is likely to elicit a response that tells you something about the wine and why you've been offered a taste. It might just be a desire to show customers something they might like. But it might also be a desire to move product that's using up space, about to go bad or just provides the seller with a higher margin. Taking your time while you taste it will give you time to consider the possibilities. Even if you decline the wine, you'll have gained some valuable information, put everyone on notice that you can taste for yourself and exhibited the most fundamental characteristic of a true connoisseur—confidence in your ability to know what you like and don't like.

I've found many sommeliers, waiters and proprietors who will knock themselves out to show you what they have. If they truly care about their wines, they've put some effort into their inventory, and are delighted to have someone who appreciates that and is willing to learn something from them about the wines they serve. On many occasions, I've received more wine for free than wine I ordered.

Can You Trust Them?

Whenever you're purchasing wine, you'll want to know whether you can trust the people selling it to you to put aside self-interest and help you find a wine that fills your needs, rather than their pockets. If you're like me, this fear can be a considerable impediment to getting a conversation started. For many years, I was certain that the moment I opened my mouth, something I said would signal my limited knowledge and expose my vulnerability to exploitation.

Sadly, these fears were not entirely unjustified. More than once, the sommelier at a well-regarded restaurant was able to intimidate me into buying, for more than I was ready to pay, an unsuitable wine. I still remember with some bitterness a few occasions when I meekly accepted a bogus recommendation simply because I didn't feel as though I knew enough to contradict it.

In retrospect, however, it was a mistake to worry about my own limited knowledge and a further mistake not to take advantage of what I did know. Daniel Webster, the famous debater, was once accused of having little knowledge of the subject he was speaking about. He confessed that his knowledge was limited, but countered that his opponent's ignorance was vast. This is useful to think about when it comes to wine.

Even professionals with encyclopedic wine knowledge will have areas they are unfamiliar with and will be concerned with how they appear to you. When I was taken advantage of, it was largely my quiet submissiveness that opened me up to manipulation. Had I simply begun to talk about what I knew, like what we were planning to order or even just how thick or thin the wine list was, I would have started a conversation that put the cunning sommelier at risk of being exposed to me or someone else nearby. That probably would have been enough to discourage a totally unsuitable recommendation.

Any conversation about purchasing wine should involve the taste of the wine, a fairly open-ended subject matter about which at this point you know much more than most people do. You may even know enough to spot a small mistake and can then judge whether it's an honest one, or an indication that something is amiss. More important, you know enough to expect a retailer or sommelier to ask you about your needs and preferences. If these aren't mentioned at all, you've a right to be suspicious.

On the other hand, it's reasonable to expect that someone who is in the business will know more about choosing a wine than you do. If you're clear about what you want to spend, what you like and what you need, you'll probably have more success taking a recommendation than choosing for yourself. If the circumstances don't permit you to mention price out loud, point to any wine in your price range and ask about it. Any real pro knows how to read that signal.

There are a number of other strategies you can employ to figure out whether you should trust someone who is selling you wine. If you don't have a reliable recommendation for a retailer or restaurant, there are telltale signs you can look for as to whether the establishment really knows what it's doing. I've already warned against restaurants that ask you to select a wine before you've had the chance to review a menu. If they don't offer you a wine list at all, it's usually best not to ask for one. In a wine shop, a prominent display in a sunny window is a troubling sign, unless the bottles are empty. Make note of the room temperature as well. Wine can deteriorate rapidly at temperatures most humans find comfortable. How the retailer deals with this is often telling. If fine wines are stored on high shelves, near radiators or otherwise exposed to temperatures above the ambient temperatures enjoyed by the staff in the shop, management might care more about being comfortable than keeping the wines in pristine condition. It's always a good sign when your local retailer wears a sweater.

Ending the Conversation

The conversation about a wine doesn't need to stop after it's been ordered. If you've been successful in ordering a good bottle, it's worth discussing with the people you're sharing it with. But be careful not to overdo it. Wine should be an integral part of a meal or an occasion. As such, it should not stand out or be the subject of undue attention. Let the conversation flow and don't push it. If the wine stimulates a great conversation about something else, it's doing its job. Leave it alone.

We all have an image of the archetypal wine bore in our mind. If you're older, the image is likely to be of a pompous, self-important windbag who thinks knowing about wine is a status symbol. Younger people will picture a compulsive wine data hound, happily swimming aimlessly in an ocean of trivial information. To my mind, a real wine bore is someone who says boring things about wine, and I actually don't think I've ever met one (although there are a few folks on the borderline). Even so, I worry that I could be a wine bore myself and I try to make it a rule not to talk with anyone about a wine after it's selected unless they bring it up themselves. Somehow, I still find plenty of people to talk to about wine.

Whether or not you talk about wine after it's served, it's still necessary to discuss it when it's being selected. If you're ordering for a group, one of your first considerations should be whether there are satisfactory wines on offer by the glass and who might be better off with that rather than sharing a bottle you've chosen. Even when you're paying for it, it can be impolite not to ask others about their preferences, what they are eating or just if they would prefer something else besides wine. When you expect someone else to pay, of course, ordering without consulting them is just plain rude.

If you've been paying attention, you also know now that one of the first things to consider when choosing a wine is the setting in which you'll enjoy it. Sharing thoughts about this with the people around you can be particularly helpful. Not everyone may feel as hot or cold as you do at the moment or be in a mood dampened by the gray and rainy weather. They can give you important clues about how you or others might feel when you actually drink the wine you're about to select.

There are many other situations where you can talk about wine in a way that's respectful and caring of the people you're with. Now that you've almost finished this book, not talking about wine is a sin you don't need to commit. You should feel comfortable with the fact that no one knows better than you what you're looking for in a wine and appreciate the uncertainty involved in making every choice, no matter how knowledgeable you are. Knowing that someone else should only collaborate with you, rather than dictate your choice, should put you at ease.

Remember that the most important conversation is the one going on between you and the wine. Through it, you can hear what the winemaker and even the vines have to say and share in the great ongoing dialog among wine lovers everywhere. As long as you take time for that conversation, you should never find yourself at a loss for words.

Drinking Too Much or Too Little

Taking care of yourself and others

Every so often, the media buzzes with a new study that, like the ones recently done on resveratrol, shows that wine contains something good for us. This shouldn't be surprising, since wine contains hundreds of different natural substances. Along with fruit flavors, wine grapes produce vitamin C (ascorbic acid) and traces of many other beneficial vitamins and minerals. Some French doctors have even been known to prescribe specific wines to ameliorate particular medical conditions, based on trace elements in those wines that are brought up from the soils in which they are grown.

Wine's reputation as a healthful elixir is undoubtedly ancient. For centuries, it was usually safer to drink than the local water and the arrival of new wine each spring must have been accompanied by a great surge in the health and well-being of the community. As it's likely to have first been made by burying grape juice underground in the autumn and digging it up in the spring, having something so enlivening emerge after it had been buried must have seemed like magic.

Now that you've learned to get more out of wine and use it in many different ways, you're likely to wonder whether it's helpful or harmful to your health. Modern medical research has indeed documented some health benefits from moderate consumption of wine. But good physicians also understand the dangers of excessive alcohol consumption and recognize that, in some cases, even a little is too much. No one should feel truly educated about wine without understanding its risks as well as its benefits.

The Influence of Alcohol

By influencing the transmission of electrical signals through the nerves that control our muscles and the synapses in our brain, alcohol acts a central nervous system depressant. It can give us a feeling of warmth and euphoria that relaxes us and is accompanied by fairly predictable physical effects. The reduction in small-muscle control caused by alcohol lowers our coordination and level of alertness. In particular, it inhibits the ability of our eyes to focus on and track moving objects, which is critical to our ability to safely operate motor vehicles and machinery.

The changes in our brain chemistry also produce noticeable, but less predictable, emotional effects that vary with the individual. In almost all of us, there is some impairment in our reasoning and memory, a reduced sense of caution and a decline in our ability to multi-task. Both good and bad emotions may become exaggerated, leading to inappropriate behavior. Persons who have tendency toward anxiety or depression may unknowingly exacerbate their symptoms by self-medicating with alcohol, without being fully aware of the effect of their changes in mood on others.

Lawyers should love alcoholic beverages even if they never drink them. They cause people to slip and fall, make tragic errors in judgment when driving, neglect their work, abuse the people who love them and even commit crimes. No wonder Rumpole of the Old Bailey loved his "Château Pomeroy's." It wasn't just a favorite beverage, it was a gold mine.

Doctors are undoubtedly frustrated by patients who seek treatment for various conditions, such as allergies, that are actually the result of stubbornly underreported use of alcohol. More serious complications can occur when concealed alcohol use aggravates conditions like a high blood pressure, heart anomalies, diabetes and liver disease or interferes with medications.

Many people are a bit bemused by the traditional medical definition of alcoholism, but you should remember that it's like a highway speed limit. There are many situations in which the speed limit seems overly cautious. But it must take into account conditions as different as night and day, wet weather and dry, new drivers and old. The effort to develop medical guidelines for alcohol usage is similarly complicated by patient underreporting and the fact that some people are much more sensitive to the effects of alcohol than others. Your own susceptibility to the adverse effects of alcohol will depend on your particular metabolism, your age, weight and the condition of your liver. Although the guidelines are meant to be conservative, they could actually be too lenient in certain situations.

Learn to understand and pay attention to the effect that alcohol has on you. Be alert to the extra work that your liver and kidneys need to do as they metabolize and flush alcohol out of your body. The drying effects of alcohol on your skin and eyes are well documented. If you see puffy dry skin and ruddy cheeks when you look in the mirror, it's a good day to lay off the sauce.

It's not just the alcohol in wine that can cause health problems. Wines may contain sulfur and other compounds that can, depending on your personal susceptibility, cause headaches, allergies, gout and other conditions. Modern medications can alleviate some of these symptoms, but they have side effects of their own. It's preferable to keep your own consumption within limits, or learn to find wines that have less of these irritants, so you don't need to rely on medications, especially since some of them don't mix well with alcohol.

Wine also contains calories and enzymes that stimulate the appetite. Here's the exception to the rule about there being a wine to match every occasion. The best wine to match a diet, or for someone who is struggling with diabetes, may be none.

Another complicating effect of alcohol is that it can become part of a cycle of dependency. You may try to overcome the effects of too many glasses of wine one night with a few extra cups of coffee or caffeinated soft drinks the next day. A few cigarettes may calm the resulting jangled nerves, but they also speed up your metabolism, so you're more likely to feel the need for a few extra glasses of wine at night to help you slow down. So the cycle continues to escalate from day to day.

Beneficial Effects

It would be wrong to conclude that wine isn't healthy for us just because alcohol can be abused, however. Numerous studies suggest that the flavonoids in red wines, such as procyanidins and quercetin, have effects that prevent the oxidation of low-density lipoproteins (otherwise known as LDL or "bad" cholesterol). This can keep them from sticking to the walls of blood vessels. These antioxidants can also protect our DNA and chase down free radicals that contribute to coronary artery disease.

In addition to the beneficial effects of red wine in ameliorating atherosclerosis, blood clots, strokes and coronary artery disease, studies have suggested that moderate consumption of the alcohol in any wine can help protect against the common cold, ulcers, gallstones and kidney stones and relieve the symptoms of stress, essential tremors and certain gastrointestinal problems.

Despite this, wine is rarely recommended as a treatment or a recommended part of daily nutrition.

In his 2003 book, *The Science of Healthy Drinking*, the journalist Gene Ford gave numerous examples of medical research and public health studies showing that moderate consumption of alcohol is healthful and argued that neo-abolitionist special interests have prevented research into, and the dissemination of information about, the health benefits of moderate alcohol consumption. One can appreciate, however, the reservations that policy makers might have about broad recommendations concerning the benefits of alcohol consumption. Just as it wouldn't be appropriate to brand wine consumption as unhealthy just because some are unable to avoid alcohol abuse, it wouldn't be appropriate to promote it as beneficial without regard to the risks it presents to some individuals and groups.

While men who are moderate drinkers have a significantly lower incidence of heart disease than their non-drinking cohorts, it's impossible to conclude from this that consumption of red wine is entirely healthful, since the benefits of reduced heart disease must be balanced against the risks of oral cancer and other alcohol-related illnesses. Most of the studies that show a link between alcohol consumption and cancers such as lung, colorectal, liver and pancreatic cancers suggest that it's only heavy drinkers who are at significantly increased risk. However, there does seem to be a measurable link between alcohol consumption and cancers of the mouth, throat, larynx and esophagus. A number of studies also suggest that women might be more susceptible than men. Particularly troublesome are recent studies where even consumption of as little as three glasses of wine a week by teen-aged women appeared to increase the risk of breast cancer significantly.

Debates will rage about whether wine is healthy or harmful, as they do about every other subject related to wine. Since there is evidence to support both views and no shortage of passionate proponents on either side, these debates will no doubt continue for a long time. It seems obvious, however, that the degree to which wine can be either healthful or harmful depends on the person and the circumstances involved. It's essential that you have candid discussions with your doctor about your consumption of alcohol and keep abreast of developing medical studies and how they may apply to you.

Test Yourself

It's important for each of us to understand how wine affects us specifically and how its effects on us may change as our bodies are affected by age or various physical conditions. In this regard, it can help you to find a way to spend some time living without alcohol every so often. You can feel confident that you're not dependent on alcohol if you can stop at will for a meaningful period without resorting to other drugs as a substitute. During this period, which should last at least a few weeks, you can observe the changes that occur and make sure that you aren't blaming other things for the effects that alcohol or other substances in your favorite wines are having on your mind and body.

The baseline feelings developed during your substance-free periods can help you better assess how the alcohol in the wine you drink affects your health and mental functioning. This personalized knowledge will be much more valuable to you than reports about the effects of alcohol in general and give you critical information that can help you to draw the line between pleasure and pain.

When you return to wine consumption after a period away, you'll find yourself more sensitive to its effects. Pay particular attention and you can learn a great deal about your normal limits and the effects alcohol and the other substances in wine can have on you. You may find that those headaches, allergies and gastric issues you're attributing to stress are ameliorated when you take a break from wine. After you resume, certain wines may trigger these symptoms while others don't. Finding lower-sulfur or less-acidic wines could help you avoid these problems in the future.

Understanding Thirst

I've also found it useful to learn to distinguish between different types of thirst. One is a physiological thirst, brought about by the natural cycles in our bodies that stimulate our fluid intake in order to provide the water our bodies consume during normal activities. Another is the dry thirst created by disruptions in the normal fluid balance due to fluid deprivation or to depletion caused by excessive perspiration, heavy respiration or other causes.

These are not the types of thirst that wine is good at quenching, since alcohol has a diuretic effect. As the famous French oenologist and philosopher of wine, Dr. Emile Peynaud, has observed, here wine "fuels the fire it is supposed to quench."

A third type of thirst, which Dr. Peynaud calls "alimentary thirst," is active when we drink for flavor and pleasure and to aid in the consumption of food. This is a thirst that wine, as a kind of liquid condiment, is well suited to satisfy. Frequently, however, when I've found myself exceeding my limits, it has been the other types of thirsts I've been trying to satisfy, with predictably bad effects. Where I've been able to think ahead and be sure that any physiological or dry thirst has been satisfied before I drink wine, I've been more successful in staying within my limits.

The Virtue of Moderation

Many philosophers over the centuries have loved wine, singing its praises like Homer's wisest man. Socrates clearly knew how to use wine to stir up a party and facilitate sparkling conversations around his table. But he and all other clear-eyed observers of the human condition have preached moderation. As Paracelsus, the legendary sixteenth-century Swiss physician, reminds us: "Wine is a food, a medicine and a poison—it's just a question of dose."

In the earlier chapters of this book, I've shown you how to inoculate yourself from taste-blindness, feverish fads and the ill effects of carelessness and quackery. Moderation in your consumption is the best way to preserve the important health benefits wine offers, which can include relaxing us and making us more sociable. By guarding against the harmful effects of alcohol, you'll keep yourself healthier and more productive, so you'll be able to afford better wine and drink more of it in the long run. You've now learned many different ways wine can give you pleasure. Keep yourself fit, so you can fully appreciate them all.

Some Parting Words

Wine's ability to lift our spirits while channeling forces drawn from deep underground has given it a special place in religious symbolism and rituals since the dawn of history. In the Caucasus region that lies between Europe and Asia, archeologists have discovered pre-historic graves containing grapevine cuttings encased in silver, indicating a belief that wine would be welcome in the next world. In Asia, carvings on Shang and Chou oracle bones, contemporaneous with the first written language, describe religious rituals involving wine, while in Europe, the ancient Greeks and Romans were famous for their Dionysian and Bacchic rites, where wines were an integral part of efforts to connect with the immortals. Medieval epics and even more modern operas chronicle the search for the Holy Grail. Even in an age where science is sometimes seen as a new religion, there are researchers trying to unlock the secrets of longevity hidden deep in wine.

While the instinct to worship wine runs deep, the religious fervor associated with it has never been connected to any fixed or immutable truth. Its pagan deities were associated with the wilder, unpredictable forces of nature. In more orthodox religions, it has served only as a medium, celebrated either as a symbol of our connection to a merciful God or reviled as a tool of Satan.

The common wine mistakes described in this book might be referred to as sins. But they don't represent transgressions of clearly defined rules, nor is wine a stern enough deity to exact stiff punishment for transgressions of its commandments. Wine understands that rules are made to be broken, that prohibition and alcohol don't mix and that sins are a product of human nature and thus inherently difficult to overcome.

You shouldn't be surprised if, long after you've read this book, you find yourself committing some of the mistakes I've described in it. It's hard to resist the instinct to imitate behaviors we see around us every day or to disentangle from a false friend, even when we know we're hurting ourselves. But as long as you're aware of your mistakes, you'll eventually find ways to make them less often and that in turn will give you more in control over the rash impulses that get you into trouble.

Some sanctimonious souls do insist that we suffer for our wine sins. They prefer more rigid strictures, the kinds that lend themselves easily to both sweeping condemnations and vigorous hairsplitting. If they were ever inclined to pick up this book, I suspect they put it down in frustration long before they reached this chapter. But I've resisted giving you hard and fast rules for many reasons, and the main one is that the most satisfying and rewarding lessons will be those you learn for yourself, by drinking wine rather than reading about it. If you've absorbed one or another of the details in this book, I hope it comes in handy at some point, but it wasn't provided so you could commit it to memory, just to illustrate the underlying dynamics that make some wine choices brilliant and others terrible mistakes.

This book was designed to help you understand those dynamics, so you can ask better questions of yourself and others. Since it would be impossible for me to give you the answers to all the thousands of questions you'll have about wine in the future, it was more important to help you recognize what the most important questions are, how to observe the subtle clues that answer them and how to get help when you need it. Most of all, I've tried to help you determine what's most pertinent to you, so you can avoid years of confusion trying to understand answers to questions that might be important only to someone else.

There is much more to learn than I've told you in this book, but the rich complexity of wine, you should now realize, is a wonder and a delight. Like train spotters or butterfly collectors, there are many people who enjoy collecting wine, but this isn't a necessary part of enjoying it; only those misguided collectors who are more intent on cataloging their wines than enjoying them should find the complexity of wine a burden. Indeed, if you find yourself more interested in collecting wine than drinking it, you're likely to be missing the point. It's just hard to stay entirely rational and truly experience all of wine's wild and hedonistic pleasures.

As long as you keep an open mind, you should be able to enjoy any glass of wine at some level. You may not finish it, but should feel a certain thrill just in discovering what you don't like about it. When you love a wine, of course, you'll want to drink it more and understand it better, but the greatest wines will dare you to classify them and pull you so close into their embrace that it's no longer possible to focus on details.

Wine's talent for easing the grip of strictly rational thought and helping you enjoy a more spontaneous existence is one of its principal talents. But hours of pleasurable quaffing won't open up its greatest pleasures for you. To get the most out of wine, you have to make an effort to understand it, but you needn't worry about how much effort is required. Learning about wine is too pleasant a journey to rush through. Just a little attention every so often will help significantly when you first start out. Take your time and learning about wine will gradually become a natural process; its rituals as instinctive as a handshake; the search for knowledge reinforced by the magical ability of wine, even as it becomes more predictable, to reveal ever more subtle and unexpected nuances. Concentration and intuition will meld into the ultimate balance to be found in wine, that which sustains you as you glide along an endless but varied wave of pleasurable experiences.

To fully appreciate wine, you must learn both what to expect and how to appreciate the unexpected. To a greater or lesser extent, some degree of predictability in taste is the goal of every winemaker. Yet winemaking starts with a natural product, grapes, and depends on a natural process, fermentation. As a result, even wines produced in the most scientifically controlled wineries exhibit some variation. In some way, whether a wine is new to you or an old favorite, there will be something a little different about the taste each time you enjoy it. That difference could be delightful or a bit disappointing. Not knowing which is what makes it exciting.

I hope you've been encouraged to embark on a lifelong exploration of the wine world. Now that you know which details to pay attention to, rather than get lost in, you should find it easier to comprehend what wine writers and reviewers get excited about. When you read about wines and wine regions, it will be easier to pay attention to the importance of grape varieties, soils and climate.

As you explore the world of wine, let the poet be your guide. Use what you read and hear to help you explore its deeper recesses, or escape them if need be. But remember that it's your own vision that will beckon you upward and serve as your final guide, the vision born when your first instinctively sensed wine's potential to fulfill your dreams.

Try not to be like the traveler who sets out to tour a country or a continent by visiting each big city for only a few days before hopping to the next. You can explore each wine variety, style or region one bottle at a time. Until you've become fully acquainted with it, the others will wait patiently, so you can move along at whatever pace suits you best. Rather than rushing through uninhabited palaces or driving from one overcrowded tourist attraction to another, take time to wander around a bit, learn a bit of the language and get to know the people.

In return for the time and attention you give to it, wine will be increasingly generous to you. When you choose them wisely and give them the respect they deserve, it is the wines themselves that will reveal their most fascinating qualities, show you how best to take pleasure from them and bless you with a small measure of heaven on earth. When you find a wine that intrigues you, make a friend of it. Let it tell you something about where it comes from. Share your likes and dislikes and see how you get along. Make mutual friends and share quiet moments. There is no reason to rush anything; you can be sure it wants to seduce you.

If some day you can visit the vineyard and meet the winemaker, your understanding of the wine will connect you both. You'll be able to stand among the vines, feel a bond with the land and channel its ancient subterranean powers. When you leave, you'll take back something more enduring than photos, museum replicas or packages of duty-free luxuries: a deeper understanding of the wine's potential, what it struggles against and what it's trying to achieve. And each year you'll receive a message, in a secret liquid code you can learn to decipher, that tells you if all is well with the places and people you've grown to love.

Each glass of wine is filled with the power to intrigue you and the potential to delight you. It is without guile and, like a sleeping infant, offers up its mysteries through its transparency. It is we, with our own hopes and fears, who complicate it. Learn to appreciate wine for what it means to you; spend time with it; help it reveal its virtues and hold it accountable for its faults. Wine will challenge you, frustrate you at times, and thrill you at others. Don't try to understand it completely, just better. Respect its unique qualities and it will open up to you and become a steady and reliable friend forever.

Appendix A

What Makes a Wine Bad?

In the long journey from vineyard to table, there are hundreds of opportunities for a wine to be mistreated. A troubling issue for many wine consumers is how to distinguish wines that are bad from wines they simply don't like. As you become more adventuresome in your choices of wines, it's important for you to be able to tell flawed wines from those that are simply inexpensive, exotic or not to your taste.

The global wine industry is well established and competitive. A battery of professionals tastes and tests wines at various stages in the production and distribution process. These include growers, winemakers, regulators, importers, distributors and retailers. In their turn, wine critics and a large and outspoken base of surprisingly knowledgeable consumers also scrutinize the industry's efforts minutely. In response, producers and distributors go to great lengths to ensure quality control and to reassure the public that their wines are sound.

Each year, legions of tasters representing importers, distributors, retailers and restaurateurs descend on the world's wineries to slurp and spit, and ferret out flaws. In order to reassure consumers that they've nothing to hide, producers open their doors to them and many even encourage visits from the general public. As a result, most of the wines available to you will be remarkably sound.

Even the highest quality wines are subject to occasional defects, however. Almost all distributors and most reputable retailers and restaurants are remarkably willing to take responsibility for serious flaws, even though many are beyond their control. It's never fair to take advantage of this by returning a bottle just because you don't like it, unless it was strongly recommended to you. But it's your right (and some would say duty) to help keep the industry on its toes by sending back a seriously flawed wine.

To some extent, what amounts to a serious flaw is a subjective judgment, so it's best not to abuse the privilege of sending a wine back. This isn't in anyone's best interest. It can make establishments less comfortable accepting returns and, consequently, consumers wary of exercising their rights. The best bottles to send back are those that have one of the few major flaws described below. If you know how to spot these, you'll be able to reject wines with confidence and do your part in maintaining the high standards of the wine industry.

Inexpensive Wines

Contrary to what many believe, most inexpensive wines are quite sound. The proof of this is that there are so many people who love wine. If you started drinking wine at a young age and didn't have wealthy parents, you probably learned to like wine despite the fact that you were drinking inexpensive bulk wines.

For a product made from something as inherently temperamental and variable as grapes, the producers of inexpensive wines do a remarkable job of efficiently delivering a consistent product, in large quantity, at a price that's readily affordable. The skills required to produce wines on an industrial scale are different from those needed to produce them in the smaller quantities associated with finer wines, but the level of skill is still considerable. Bulk wine producers may not use the most prestigious grape varieties or grow them in the finest locations, but that's part of what makes their product inexpensive.

What distinguishes inexpensive wines from other wines isn't likely to be flaws in the wine. In fact, in large-scale production, chemicals (typically sulfur compounds) and various processes such as filtration are used to control the bacteria that can cause the most serious flaws. Since the wines are made for consumption at a very young age, screw caps and other nonporous closures can be used, ensuring that the wine does not evolve in the bottle, reaching you in much the same condition it was in when it left the winery, despite being jostled and overheated along the way.

What is sacrificed in the effort to bring a satisfactory wine to your table inexpensively is complexity and intensity in taste. The productive grape varieties used and the way the grapes are grown maximize volume, while the chemicals and filtration strip away flavor elements. Large-scale, mechanized harvesting and the use of less-optimal sites reduce the chances that the grapes will be at the peak of ripeness and flavor when they are delivered to the winery. The result is wines that have a narrow range of flavors and are less likely to resonate with the fairly wide range of flavors in a typical meal.

It's the search for more vibrant and interesting flavors that sets most wine lovers off in search of better wines and makes it worth it to pay more, sometimes much more, for them. A well-known premium wine can command a price at least three or four times the price of the average bulk wine, but there is large quantity of wine priced in the no-man's land between these price levels. Some of these are simply bulk quality wines named and packaged to simulate premium wine or, alternatively, given a fresh and arresting label to look like something new and different. Others were made to be premium wines and fell victim to one or more of the many minor flaws in the winemaking process.

There are many relatively unknown producers, however, who are working hard to make premium wines and succeed to a greater or lesser degree from year to year. Their wines often can be as good or better than others that sell for many multiples of their price. Once you learn how to find them and where to use them, these less expensive wines will serve their purpose at least as well as an expensive wine would. Bear in mind that many of the factors that increase the cost of producing an expensive wine relate to preparing it for cellaring. Unless you have a reason to drink a well-aged wine, a wine that's been made to be drunk earlier will be more suitable, and you shouldn't have to pay nearly as much for it.

Premium Wines

When producers make an effort to preserve and enhance the natural flavors in their wines, many of the practices they follow increase the opportunities for flaws to arise. Reducing reliance on pesticides, irrigation, filtration and aggressive sulfur treatments, while increasing reliance on skin contact, wild yeasts and slow fermentation, significantly increases the opportunity for harmful bacteria and mold to enter the wine. Diligent and costly efforts can substantially reduce, but never completely eliminate, these risks.

This creates a bit of a quandary for the consumer, who is both paying more for the wine and taking a greater risk that it will be flawed. Learning how to spot these flaws can give you more confidence that an investment in a more expensive bottle is worth the price, because you'll feel comfortable returning it when that's appropriate.

The most common and easily recognized flaws in wine are heat damage, cork taint and premature oxidation. The causes and effects of these problems are described briefly below. Don't expect to find them in many bottles. When you do find them, however, it's your right to bring it the attention of whoever sold you the bottle and expect to receive a refund or a new bottle in exchange. Think of what you paid for the wine as including a premium to insure your right to make the return.

Heat Damage

Heat damage frequently goes unnoticed because it's fairly common and consumers simply confuse the effects with attributes of poorly made wines they don't like. This is a pity because it not only can give a good wine a bad name, it can make an establishment complacent about the one problem it can do the most to correct, by ensuring that its wines are properly stored.

High heat accelerates the processes that deteriorate a wine. In a bottle with a firm closure, such as a screw cap, this can lead to reductive collapse, where the flavors are essentially cooked into oblivion. When a bottle with a more porous closure, such as a cork, is subject to extremes of temperature, pressure differentials can speed the flow of oxygen through the bottle and accelerate oxidation and bacterial growth.

Even a bottle of wine several decades old will exhibit a certain freshness in taste if it was made to age and properly stored. If you drink a bottle of wine that is less than ten years old and it tastes vinegary, dry and flavorless, it has been damaged either by exposure to extreme heat for a limited period of time (sometimes only a few hours is enough) or by extended storage in a warm place.

There is a limit to how long any wine can be safely stored. Wines older than thirty are best purchased as collector's items and not for consumption. You may be able to taste them as a novelty, but shouldn't expect them to be great wines, regardless of the price they can command.

Cork Taint

Cork taint is caused by Tyrene (trichloroanisole or TCA), a compound that smells like a warm, damp old cellar inhabited by wet newspapers, sofas and dirty dogs. It's caused by various filamentous fungi that create Tyrene as a byproduct of ingesting chlorine and bromine related compounds. These can creep into improperly made corks or take up residence in the wine directly due to inattentive sanitary practices in the winery. Tyrene is highly irritating (a few teaspoons would be sufficient to spoil all the wine made in France), but it can take a bit of time, and more than one sip, for you to notice it.

Whenever you sniff a wine and there is an earthiness that suggests a bit of mold, you should take extra care in tasting the wine. Sip it more than once and let some time pass. There are earthy tastes in wine that can suggest an unpleasant moldiness at first, but these usually dissipate to leave a delicious wine. If there is Tyrene in the wine, however, the moldy taste will persist and become increasingly annoying.

When you're tasting a wine in a restaurant you may feel pressure to make a decision before you can decide whether there is cork taint or not. When this happens, it's customary to mention to the server that you think the bottle might be suffering from cork taint and invite someone from the establishment to take a small taste. By the time they do, you can usually be sure.

It's not usually necessary to order a completely different wine when you detect a bottle that's affected by cork taint. Most of the time, for older wines, it's only the odd bottle that's been affected and you can ask for another bottle of the same wine with some confidence that it won't be afflicted by the same condition. When a younger wine is tainted, however, it can be a sign that the condition was allowed to build up during the winemaking process and other bottles from the same winery and vintage are more likely to have been affected.

Excessive Oxidation

Some oxidation occurs naturally in all wines and some, such as Madeira, Sherry and various "yellow wines" are deliberately oxidized in order to bring out nutty, sweet and sour flavors. Most wines, however, need to be protected from excessive oxidation, which can flatten out the color, aroma and flavor in a wine, as oxygen binds with the phenols and ethanols in the wine that give it brightness and fruity flavors.

Any well-aged wine will show some signs of oxidation in the form of a brown rim in the glass and a slight increase in richness and sweetness. This comes from the gradual breakdown of citric acid, which is usually not found in great quantity in wines that are made to age. However, excessive exposure to oxygen during or after the fermentation process, abnormally high heat levels during storage and other causes can create a more pronounced buildup of acetic acid and begin to turn any wine into vinegar. When it reaches a level of above 600 mg/L, it gets offensive to most people.

You may, at some point, become so intrigued by what an old wine might taste like that you'll purposely purchase a vinegary wine. The person who sells it to you should be aware of the likelihood that the wine will be oxidized and warn you. If they do, you can't blame them for the condition of the wine. But you can blame them if it's not reasonably priced. Other than deliberately oxidized wines like Sherry and Madeira, or legendary old wines sold to collectors who never drink them, wines that are oxidized should not be sold to consumers. Someone in the delivery chain should have weeded them out.

If you're not warned about the possibility of excessive oxidation and notice a pronounced brownish color in your wine, be on the alert. In some cases, you may find it decidedly pleasant or only mildly distracting. But if you notice a pronounced taste of vinegar, the wine is bad and you're entitled to a refund.

Appendix B

Major Grape Varieties

Only a very small percentage of the many grape varieties identified by botanists are in the genus *Vitis vinifera*. And of the hundreds of varieties within that genus, only a handful are used to produce most of the wine consumed in the world today. The varieties described below have been chosen to provide a worthy sampler for your consideration, and also because they're used to make wines that are readily available around the world today. The listing is by no means complete.

Chardonnay and Cabernet Sauvignon can be logical varieties to start with as you first begin to explore the characteristic tastes different grape varieties impart to the wines made from them. Since they're widely available, you're at least likely to be somewhat familiar with them, even if neither of them ends up being a particular favorite of yours. What's more important is that each represents a different challenge you can overcome as you proceed to master the art of tasting wine in a discriminating way.

Chardonnay's challenge is that it's extremely adaptable, and exhibits different characteristics depending on where it's grown. The differences in taste, however, reflect those that climate has on wines in general. So in learning to identify Chardonnay, you'll be introducing yourself to tastes that will be reprised when you move on to other varieties and you'll be able appreciate them as being influenced by climate rather than grape variety. Many, but not all of the wines made from Chardonnay are aged in oak. As one of the few white wines readily available in both oaked and un-oaked versions, it can also provide a good example of the qualities oak aging can impart to a wine. This ability to provide insights into the differences that both geography and winemaking style can impart to wine makes Chardonnay a particularly good place to start learning about the characteristic tastes of wine.

Cabernet Sauvignon presents a completely different challenge. It tastes very similar to other frequently used varieties, such as Merlot and Cabernet Franc. Learning what distinguishes Cabernet Sauvignon from these other varieties is an exercise in the subtler distinctions that can make a wine unique.

Experienced wine tasters may find my grouping of wine varieties by fruit taste a bit controversial. One can rarely describe accurately the taste of the wines produced from a particular wine variety by associating it with one specific fruit taste. The flavors in the wines made from any single variety will vary significantly depending on where the grapes are grown and how the wine is made. Each person will also tend to experience different flavors based on the particularities of his or her own palate. As a result, many descriptions of wine by variety are not specific about the fruit flavors. Similarly, groupings of wines in many wine books are often made by region or according to such characteristics as "body" or even price.

Most beginners, however, seem to find the broad progression from citrus to spice used below useful in organizing their initial thoughts about grape varietals and the tastes they can be expected to exhibit. The categories I've used are those that seem to create taste expectations broad enough to include the majority of wines made from the varieties listed in each category, yet narrow enough to be distinguishable from the varieties in the other categories. I am, of course, assuming that you'll be prepared for the inevitable exceptions and alert for the impact that stylistic factors have on the finished product.

In general, for both the reds and the whites, the groups listed tend to progress from varieties produced in cooler areas to those produced in warmer areas. As a result, the progression will tend to move from lighter-bodied wines where the fruit flavors are subtler and acidity is more evident, to heavier wines with bolder, spicier flavors and a higher alcohol content. With both the whites and the reds, wines at the end of the first grouping or the beginning of the second will sometimes exhibit fruit qualities that would make them suitable to be included in the other group. Thus, to keep things simple as you build an appreciation of the differing qualities of red and white wines, I suggest you start your investigations with varieties at the beginning of the list of whites and toward the end of the list of reds.

Some will ask why there is no listing of rosé wine varieties. The reason is not that there are no grape varieties particularly associated with rosé wines, but that there are so many of them, and so few of them are used exclusively to make any significant quantity of rosé wine. In general, the varieties that are used almost exclusively to make rosé are used only as a small part of the overall mix and even the wines that contain them are relatively rare. Those rosés that are produced in quantity are generally made principally from red wine grapes that have either been harvested early or made so that the juice is given limited contact with the pigment-producing skins. Where rosé versions of a red wine grape are helpful to understanding the characteristics of the variety, they are mentioned below.

Bear in mind that this listing isn't intended to simply catalog various grape varieties and their characteristics, but to help you learn to identify the flavors that these common grape varieties bring to a wine. This will help you develop an even deeper understanding of the characteristics that are imparted to a wine by climate and the stylistic choices of the winemaker.

Citrus Fruit Whites

Sauvignon Blanc makes crisp, nervy wines with an aggressive bite. There is a clean, bitter edge and dry texture to Sauvignon Blanc that is reminiscent of wild vegetables and herbs. Thus the name, which translates as "wild white." The fruit taste is usually reminiscent of unripe apples or plums or the tartest of grapefruits, while the herbal notes can suggest mint, basil and fresh-cut grass or hay. Wines made from Sauvignon Blanc are very aromatic and are among the easiest to identify by aroma alone, as they usually give off a characteristic whiff of ammonia and smoke. They are typically consumed at a lower temperature than other wines, and are usually made in a fresh and fruity style that rewards immediate consumption. This makes them good bets to quench your thirst during warm weather. Because they rarely benefit from extended fermentation or storage in wood, Sauvignon Blancs can be produced less expensively and are often targeted to the price conscious market. However, those from areas with deep chalky soils can exhibit steely, flinty mineral flavors and aromas suggestive of gun smoke and can sometimes benefit from extended cellaring. In other areas, the wines can be either stonier or more delicate and are sometimes made as sweeter, late-harvest wines. Sauvignon Blanc is the staple white grape of Bordeaux, where is it usually blended with wine made from the much sweeter and fuller variety, Semillon, to make wines that are unctuous, but still have a defined edge. Because of their lively herbaceous flavors and crisp acidity, wines made from Sauvignon Blanc often make a good match with vegetarian dishes, particularly those that feature bitter herbs, and also do well with fried chicken, grilled fish and oysters. It's one of the few wines that have a hope of matching with green asparagus and is a particular favorite with sharp cheeses, such as the soft cheeses made with goat's milk. Iconic versions of the flintier style are made from grapes grown on the steep hillsides of Sancerre and Pouilly-Fumé along the banks of the Loire River, while leading producers in the Graves area of the Médoc make the most legendary Sauvignon Blanc/Semillon blends. Outstanding examples of Sauvignon Blanc are also produced in New Zealand, northern California, northeastern Italy and Slovenia. In Germany and Austria, Sauvignon Blanc is referred to as Muskat-Silvaner, while in the United States, South Africa, Australia and New Zealand it's often referred to as Fumé Blanc.

Chardonnay is popular because it gets around. It can be found in almost every wine-producing region. The wines in each region have a following even though they can taste markedly different. The basic fruit flavors range widely from white peaches and pears in cooler, higher-latitude areas, to melons and even decidedly tropical tastes like pineapple, banana, guava and mango in warmer, lower-latitude areas. Wines made from Chardonnay can range from crisp and fresh to rich and opulent and from light and sparkling to full-bodied and austere. As a grape variety, Chardonnay can provide a match for many different foods and occasions, but what matches with it will depend on the style of the wine made from it. Chardonnays made in the French style, emphasize minerality and pair well with simply prepared white meat and fish dishes. Those made in a more fruit-forward style are full-bodied enough to stand up to oriental spices and other strongly flavored food. Named for a town in Burgundy, it's a genetic cousin of Pinot Noir, and is well known as the signature Burgundian white grape, although there are small quantities of wine produced from at least four other white grape varieties in Burgundy. Champagne made exclusively from Chardonnay is labeled "Blanc de Blanc" to distinguish it from the more common Champagnes made from Pinot Noir or a blend of grapes. Many new-world sparkling wines are also made from Chardonnay. Iconic versions of Chardonnay are the very different Grand Cru wines of Chablis and the Côte de Beaune in Burgundy and the wines from producers such as Château Montelena and Grgich Hills in Napa Valley. There are notable Chardonnays produced in such diverse locations as Czech Republic, Lebanon and Canada. Although it has been given about two dozen different names in the various wine regions of Europe, the use of these names is dying out and it's rarely referred to by any other name in the rest of the world.

Riesling makes crisp, light-bodied wines of honeyed delicacy. Many people tend to think of Rieslings as sweet wines and are surprised when wine professionals refer to a wine made from Riesling as a dry or acidic wine. However, many Rieslings are low in alcohol, which itself tastes sweet at lower concentrations and creates a satisfying counterbalance for their acidity even when they have little residual sugar. These everyday Rieslings don't display the syrupy sweetness associated with dessert wines (although many late-harvest Rieslings are among the most renowned dessert wines). Their evident acidity allows them to pair well with fish, vegetables and other light to medium-bodied foods. They are particular favorites with fried foods: fish and chips in Britain and schnitzels in Germany and Austria. The inherent sweetness of the variety is on particular display in the wines made in the Northern Rhine and Mosel river valleys in Germany, where official definitions of quality depend on the level of residual sugar. Many German and Austrian producers have offerings at escalating levels of sweetness, from Kabinett (the driest) to Spätlese and various categories of Auslese (the sweetest) and reserve their best grapes for the sweeter wines. These grapes will produce not only the green apple, lemon, lime and white peach type fruit flavors characteristically associated with Riesling, but also strong minerality and a certain hint of oiliness (a whiff of a scent surprisingly like benzene). Since Rieslings are prized for their delicate aromatics, they're often served in small rounded glasses to minimize the amount of air contact once they are poured. The aromatics are improved with age, but decanting even a young Riesling would be controversial. The mineral qualities are emphasized and the residual sugar reduced in wines produced from Riesling in the Alsace region of France. These sturdier wines pair well with honey-glazed baked hams and various other fresh, cured or smoked pork products, as well as sauerkraut and onion tarts. There are many outstanding producers of Riesling in the Rhine and Mosel valleys and in Alsace. Notable Rieslings are also made in Austria and northern Italy and in South Africa's Cape region. Good Rieslings are also made in the Willamette Valley in Oregon and the Finger Lakes region of New York in the United States as well as the Barossa area of Australia. There are many variations on the name of the variety, most of which contain the word Riesling or something that sounds like it. Unfortunately, there was a time when producers in Australia and California used the name Riesling to refer to any fruity white wine, which gave the variety a bad name it may not yet have recovered from.

Tropical Fruit Whites

Pinot Grigio is one of Italy's best-known varieties. Called **Pinot Gris** in Alsace and several other names in France, it appears under the name **Ruländer** and others in Germany, Switzerland, Austria, Hungary, Slovakia and Romania. Like its cousin Chardonnay, it exhibits markedly different characteristics as it travels, so different in fact, that it seems to mutate into an entirely different grape, although in all regions it produces wines with a refreshing, vibrant fruitiness. Flavors can range from delicately clean white melons to apricots with hints of nuts and honey. The Italian wines produced from Pinot Grigio are light and acidic, which makes them suitable for pairing with lighter pasta dishes and simply prepared fish and chicken dishes. In Germany and other countries along the Danube, Pinot Grigio makes a full-bodied white that is a bit lower in acidity, yet carries a hint of spiciness in the aroma. Here the relationship with Chardonnay seems most obvious. In Alsace, the grapes are typically picked earlier to preserve their acidity and are both spicier and lighter in body than their German counterparts. Alsatian Pinot Gris tends to be made in a heavier, sweeter style that pairs well with sausages and many spicy Asian preparations. The best Pinot Grigios in Italy tend to come from the northeastern regions of Alto Adige and Friuli, while in Germany outstanding examples are produced in the Baden and Pfalz wine-growing regions. Every leading wine producer in Alsace will have premium offerings of Pinot Gris.

Chenin Blanc provides a study in structure. It makes wines that range from the austerely dry to the lusciously sweet, yet its vibrant acidity can infuse a wine with zest and incredible longevity and give unexpected lightness to even its thickest and richest expressions. Called **Steen** in South Africa, it is the most widely planted variety and its fresh fruitiness is emphasized, while in France's Loire Valley, where it first established itself as capable of making leading world-class wines, the emphasis is on longevity. In areas like Vouvray and Saumur along the Loire, Chenin Blancs are made in a variety of styles ranging from sophisticated sparking wines to unctuous dessert wines. Producers typically offer a range of still wines from early-drinking, racy dry wines to sweeter, more age-worthy wines that can take several decades to reach their peak. In between gushing youth and glorious old age, Chenin Blancs typically experience a painful and difficult adolescence, during which they become nasty and foul-tasting. This undoubtedly accounts for the aversion many wine drinkers have to them, as well as the feeling among their many passionate proponents that they are misunderstood. Genetically descended from Sauvignon Blanc, Chenin Blanc provides a similarly high level of acidity and produces wines with a similar lightness and crispness, while providing flavors that are rounder and more suggestive of pears, apples, quinces and even tropical fruits, often with hints of almonds. The combination of roundness and crispness allows the sparkling wines to pair well with cream sauces, pâté and other rich dishes. The drier style still wines can pair well with salads, fish, chicken and other light dishes. Somewhat sweeter Chenin Blancs can provide a spectacular match for curry and other spicy dishes.

Gewürztraminer is a wine with complicated origins and complex tastes. There is not a great deal of it produced, but it's usually a crowd pleaser. Gewürztraminer means "spicy traminer" and is believed to have originated in Switzerland. Various clones of it are still grown there and in Germany, but it's a difficult grape to grow and seems best suited to the sloping foothills of Alsace in France. While it can be too unsubtle for some people, most who try it enjoy its exotic rose petal bouquet and cascade of spicy ginger, honeysuckle, citrus and tropical-fruit flavors. It often reminds people of lychee nuts and, as a low-acid wine, is a natural choice with spicy Asian cuisine. Although genetically unrelated to two other Alsatian varieties, Pinot Blanc and Pinot Gris, it's customary to think of them as a progression in terms of the fragrance and spiciness of their flavors, with Gewürztraminer considered to be a version of Pinot Gris on steroids.

Viognier makes complicated and powerful wines; so powerful and fragrant that they are sometimes blended in to brighten up hearty reds. In the northern Rhône Valley, talented growers and winemakers produce oily, seductive wines from Viognier that have a signature taste of spicy apricots, along with grilled nuts and a host of other subtle flavors. It's a difficult variety to grow, however, and hasn't traveled extensively outside the Rhône region. Recently, winemakers in cooler areas of California and Australia have produced some promising Viogniers.

Other White Pinots – While most grape varieties are rather indiscriminate in their mating habits, the Pinot family can be downright degenerate. Crossings and mutations abound, some of which distinguish themselves sufficiently to gain recognition as separate varieties. Within the extended family are a number of Chardonnay descendants, such as Aligote, Auxerrois, Melon and Beaunoir, all of which taste similar to Chardonnay, but have sufficiently distinctive characteristics to merit a niche of their own. (Most are grown in areas where Chardonnay is also grown and it can be fun to taste them side by side with Chardonnay to see if you can pick out the subtle yet significant differences yourself.) The Pinot family contains several mutations of Pinot Noir whose grapes produce colors ranging from the cloudy blue of Pinot Gris to pinkish-white, although their genetic structure is almost identical to Pinot Noir. Aside from Pinot Gris, the most notable are Pinot Blanc, which can exhibit a wonderful blend of floral aromas and stony minerality, and Pinot Meunier, a secret ingredient in many types of Champagne. Pinot Meunier is valued for its ability to add body and fruitiness while at the same time bringing lighter color and crisper acidity to many nonvintage Champagne blends. Like Pinot Gris and Pinot Blanc, Pinot Meunier has found a home in various wine regions around the world, particularly in Germany, Switzerland and Austria, where it's used to make red wine and known variously as Schwarzriesling, Müllerrebe and Müller-Traube. More recently, Pinot Meunier has been planted in Australia and New Zealand. In California, Melon de Bourgogne, the variety used to make the ubiquitous Muscadets served in the bistros of Paris, was once thought to be a variety of Pinot Blanc, but it has been identified as a cross between Pinot Blanc and Gouais Blanc. Planted near the ocean, it has a remarkable ability to pick up the salty taste of the sea breezes, which makes Muscadet a great alternative to Sauvignon Blanc and Chardonnay as a combination with oysters and other shellfish.

Other Rhône Whites – The Rhône Valley also produces some arrestingly different wines from the Marsanne and Roussanne grape varieties. Although more often blended with other grapes to make rosé or even red wines, these grapes can produce some very interesting wines on their own. Marsanne can produce a clear, high-alcohol white wine with emerald green flashes that looks like it should be austerely dry, while the aromas are fruity and flowery and remind many of honeysuckle with a whiff of glue. While young, the wines have nectarine-like tastes, but are crisp and deliciously dry. With aging, however, wines made from early-picked grapes can grow in complexity, adding a bit of sweetness and a golden brown color. By contrast, Roussanne has a citrusy edge to it and gives off more delicate aromas. Undoubtedly for this reason, it is primarily used in blends, often with Marsanne, where it adds herbal notes.

Red-Fruit Reds

Pinot Noir is believed by many Burgundy lovers to be the only red grape you'll ever need. Passionate Pinotphiles justify these claims by pointing to the remarkable ability of the variety to express subtle differences in soil and microclimate in pronounced ways. Small communes in Burgundy have learned over the centuries how to showcase these differences and produce a remarkably diverse collection of wines that range from light to medium-bodied and exhibit fruit flavors that range from delicate raspberries to black cherries. It's fortunate that the variety lends itself to such diversity, because it does not travel nearly as well as its cousin Chardonnay. Although there are choice locations in Germany, Italy, New Zealand, California and Oregon where the variety can produce extraordinary wines, it's notoriously hard to grow and winemakers often struggle to make decent wine from the grape even in Burgundy. This is one variety for which knowing the good years can make the difference between a wine that is supple and satisfying and one that is thin and sharp. The combination of intense flavor and moderate levels of acidity and alcohol make Pinot Noirs particularly food-friendly. The variety of fruit flavors, floral aromas and earthy undertones that the wines exhibit allows them to provide matches for everything from oysters to beef and game. In Burgundy, iconic Pinot Noirs of substance are produced from the Grand Cru vineyards of Vosne-Romanée, while graceful and hauntingly delicate wines can be produced from the premier cru and grand cru vineyards of Volnay and Chambolle-Musigny. Remarkable wines are produced from Pinot Noir in Santa Barbara county and the Russian River area of California and along the Willamette River in Oregon. These tend to be new-world wines, however, with less earthiness, higher alcohol levels and sweeter fruit. Most Pinot Noir wines are consumed within the first seven or eight years, but the sturdier Burgundies can take decades to reach their peak.

Garnacha isn't easy to find as a red wine in its pure form, because producers almost uniformly blend it with wine from other grapes. Late to ripen, it's well adapted to warmer wine regions and tolerates stony soils and winds that few other vines would survive. While it can provide flavors ranging from raspberry or pomegranate to plum, its main virtue is as a base for many notable blends. Its low acidity softens the austere, tannic tastes of wines made from other warm climate grape varieties, and its high alcohol level can unlock their fragrances. Garnacha is the most widely planted variety in Spain, and is a contender for that honor in France and Australia as well, where it's typically known as **Grenache**. It's also a major variety in California, in Sardinia and Sicily in Italy, and in countries as diverse as Lebanon, South Africa and Morocco. Garnacha is the principal variety in most Rioja wines, where it's blended with Tempranillo. It's also the principal grape in the wines from Châteauneuf-du-Pape, Gicondas and other areas in France's Rhône Valley, where it's blended with Syrah and numerous other varieties. Wines made exclusively from Garnacha can be found in the Priorat and Navarra regions of Spain, but these are not necessarily indicative of the tastes that are contributed to the blends, since the grapes are much more restricted in yield. This results in grapes that produce more color, higher acidity and less alcohol, and fruit flavors that can be more reminiscent of darker fruit. One can get a better sense of what the variety contributes to a blend by drinking one of the many rosé wines that are made exclusively from Garnacha. These wines typically rely on grapes grown to maximize their productivity and do not depend on dark skins to produce their flavors. Because of the ability of the varieties it's blended with to dominate, these varieties will often be more important factors in determining which foods the wines match best with, even when Garnacha is the dominant component by volume.

Gamay is to some extent a victim of its own success. It is almost exclusively associated with the wines of the Beaujolais region of France and is popular for its ability to make wines that are highly quaffable when young. Made in an easily produced, ready to drink style, notably as "Beaujolais Nouveau," the wines have enough acidity to be thirst-quenching and are inexpensive enough to use as everyday wines. These wines are good to get to know if you're on a hamburger and hot dog food budget, but they lack a bit in style. While most of the Beaujolais region has embraced and exploited the easygoing virtues of the variety, there are still dedicated producers in the ten small areas designated to produce "Cru Beaujolais" wines, who succeed in producing something more age-worthy and refined. These are a diverse group of wines ranging from the chillingly ethereal Chiroubles to the warm, dense Morgons that express the granitic soils of the region with distinction. Chilling these wines would be a mistake, although it can be quite appropriate for their lesser siblings. It's a sign of the innate character of Gamay that for many years some California growers apparently confused it with a particular strain of Pinot Noir. Deep red with purple highlights, the wines typically exhibit flavors of strawberries and raspberries, sometimes with a hint of vanilla that suggests bananas.

Sangiovese is the dominant grape variety grown in Tuscany and, as an officially recommended variety in 53 provinces, is the most widely planted grape in Italy. It's been the principal component in Chianti for generations and, with the cooperation of climate change and more rational regulations, is increasingly emerging from the blend to stand on its own in many single variety Chianti Classicos. The success of wines made purely from clones such as Brunello in Montalcino or Prugnolo in Montepulciano has encouraged producers to search for the clones suitable for making single varietal wines in other areas of the region. At the same time, there has been a movement to blend Sangiovese with black fruit varieties like Merlot and Cabernet Sauvignon to produce more "modern" wines that have more global appeal. While some Sangiovese has been planted for many years in Argentina and several producers have experimented with it in California, there is little Sangiovese planted outside Italy. A characteristic of Sangiovese is its acidity. It produces high levels of durable tartaric acid that persist even in the warmer years and help make the wines long lasting. Italians tend to like tannic, bitter tastes in their wines, and wines made from Sangiovese in the traditional style tend to exhibit bitter black cherry and herbal notes. The preference for bitterness has conveniently allowed the *riserva* wines (those made for the long haul) to be aged in Slovenian oak, which does not impart as much of a woody flavor and sweetness to the wines, although they will display hints of vanilla. Don't be afraid to decant or otherwise aerate even a middle-aged *riserva*; they often taste even better in the morning. Sangiovese is often paired with simply grilled meats prepared with herbs, particularly veal chops and steaks, and its acids also work well with pasta dishes that feature tomato sauces. In addition to Prugnolo and Brunello, there are numerous other names used for Sangiovese and its various clones, some that include Sangiovese in the name and others that don't, such as Morellino, Calabrese, Nerino and Sanvicetro.

Cabernet Franc is lean and green. It's the earliest ripening of the legendary triumvirate of Bordeaux blends: Cabernet Franc, Merlot and Cabernet Sauvignon. That it has a life of its own is amply demonstrated. The revered wines of Château Cheval Blanc in St. Émilion rely heavily and at times exclusively on Cabernet Franc. In addition, the wines of Bourgueil and Chinon in the Loire Valley, which are made exclusively from Cabernet Franc, can be long lasting and exceptional in their own right, although quite different from Cheval Blanc. Wines made exclusively from Cabernet Franc are more aggressively herbaceous than those made from Cabernet Sauvignon. It can add accents of blueberries to Bordeaux blends, while the Bourgueils are characterized by notes of dark cherries and strawberries and the Chinons by softer red berries. They tend to be excellent matches with roasted meats, especially pork, and also have an affinity for eggplant. Despite the predominance of red fruit flavors, Cabernet Franc can taste remarkably similar to Cabernet Sauvignon and Merlot, and when blended with them can appear to add little to the overall result. Its main function may be to serve as a hedge against cool weather, and provide color and a measure of herbaceousness when the Cabernet Sauvignon hasn't had the opportunity to fully ripen. Because of its hardiness in cool weather, Cabernet Franc is planted widely in Eastern Europe and northern Italy, where it's sometimes referred to as "Bordo."

Dark Fruit Reds

Barbera is capable of producing great wines, but often used as a filler, prized more for its hot-weather reliability and productivity than its taste. When well made, however, it can produce a stunning wine with bracing acidity and lots of tarry, mouth-filling fruit, such as blackberries, black cherries and plums. It works well with roasted meats and stews, and it makes it a classic companion to cream of mushroom soup. Few Barbera wines are made to age, but they will benefit from time in the glass, and those made for the long haul can be something of a revelation. In Italy, the grape seems to be best suited to the hills around Alba in the Piedmont, where it has serious competition from Nebbiolo, which can produce more profitable wines. In California, Argentina, Uruguay, Brazil and other areas of Italy, it's used mostly as a filler to improve the acid or alcohol level of the final product.

Nebbiolo produces the renowned Barolos and Barbarescos of the Piedmont in Italy, where the patient producers of the Lange region use it to make long-lasting wines of extraordinary nobility whose pronounced but delicate aromas remind some of roses or violets, while others make a natural association with Piedmont's legendary black truffles. The wines can provide a battery of flavors including black cherry, mulberry, licorice, tar, tobacco, pepper and leather. The array of flavors makes the wines suitable for matching with an array of foods, but because of the heavy tannin levels, they work best with meaty risottos and other rich, heavily flavored meat, fish and pasta dishes. In addition to Barolo and Barbaresco, Nebbiolo is used in the northern Italy to make a table wine under the name of Spanna, and is used in several blends of only local significance. It's rarely cultivated outside of Italy.

Merlot is a both a workhorse and a show horse in the Bordeaux region of France and has displayed its talents as both partner and prince in other wine regions as well. It plays only a supporting role in many of the sought-after blends from the Médoc area in Bordeaux, where the renowned "first growths" feature Cabernet Sauvignon, Cabernet Franc and other varieties. But Merlot is used exclusively for almost all of the other red wines produced in the region, including the famous "right bank" wines of St. Émilion and Pomerol, where the iconic Petrus, Le Pin and L'Evangile wines are produced. Merlot is famous for producing a riotous array of tastes. It sometimes displays pronounced red berry flavors, but they seem roasted and it's often described as "plummy." It also will display vegetal tastes; more like garden vegetables and not as wild as those in Cabernet Sauvignon. Known for having an aroma that often hints of violets, Merlot's signature is lower acidity, which gives it a rounder feeling, and an earthiness that many describe as giving it "animal" tastes. Its ability to pair with the ground beef in frankfurters and hamburgers is undoubtedly what makes it a favorite by-the-glass offering in bars. But these distinctions from Cabernet Sauvignon or Cabernet Franc are not as dramatic as they may seem when you hear them described. Although it's often referred to as being softer than the other Cabernet varieties, you're likely to enjoy it more if you resist the urge to quaff it down and instead let it sit in the glass a bit. When you first compare them, Merlot and Cabernet Sauvignon wines are likely to seem more similar than different, especially when made from fully ripened grapes. Some of the perceived differences may simply be attributable to which ripens earlier, but it does seem that Cabernet Franc, Merlot and Cabernet Sauvignon represent something of a progression from more red-berry tastes to more blackberry tastes, with Merlot having the capacity to exhibit elements of both. Merlot continues to grow in popularity in France and is widely planted in Italy (where it has a following independent of its role in the Super-Tuscan blends), in Slovenia and in Hungary, where it forms a part of the popular blend known as "Bull's Blood."

Cabernet Sauvignon is the long-distance champion of grape varieties. Among the latest varieties to ripen, it can produce grapes with the high levels of tannin conducive to making an age-worthy wine that will soak up cedar and other woody flavors when given time to mature in oak barrels. It also produces wines that have staying power in the mouth; a long aftertaste is the hallmark of a wine made with Cabernet Sauvignon. As the "sauvignon" in the name suggests, the French prize the "wild" vegetal tastes in Cabernet Sauvignon, undoubtedly passed down from its genetic parent Sauvignon Blanc. However, these should not be confused with a more intense garden vegetable taste, more reminiscent of bell peppers, caused by the use of under-ripe grapes, which can overwhelm the basic dark cherry, blackberry and black currant tastes in the wine. Rather, where the grapes have been properly ripened, the herbaceous elements will impart a more refined and minty quality to the younger wines (sometimes enhanced by shrewd owners who plant eucalyptus trees near the vineyard). When the wines are given time to age, the spicy, minty and cedary flavors in the wine all seem to interact to produce a refreshing, slightly watery finish that gently cleanses the palate. It would be misleading to say that there is an old-world style of Cabernet Sauvignon, since the old-world wines that feature Cabernet Sauvignon are all blends dominated (in bulk if not in taste) by other varietals. These include the iconic "first growths" of the Médoc: Lafite, Latour, Margaux, Haut Brion and Mouton. Perhaps the closest one might get to an old-world example of a pure Cabernet Sauvignon is the relative newcomer, Sassicaia, from the Bolgheri area of Tuscany, which contains only 15 percent of its close cousin Cabernet Franc. But there are many examples of extraordinary wines made exclusively from Cabernet Sauvignon in new-world wine regions such as Napa Valley and Paso Robles in California, the Columbia Valley in eastern Washington in the United States, the Maipo Valley in Chile and the Coonawarra, Margaret River and Barossa Valley areas of Australia. In the Penedès area of Spain, there are producers such as Bodegas Torres who produce new-world style wines made exclusively from Cabernet Sauvignon. Legendary Cabernet Sauvignons are produced in areas of the Napa Valley, California, such as Rutherford and the Stag's Leap, Diamond Mountain, Howell Mountain, Mt. Veeder and Spring Mountain districts. Because of its worldwide popularity, efforts are being made to plant Cabernet Sauvignon in almost every wine region. Outside of a few small areas of France, where it can be called Vidure or Bouchet, it's referred as Cabernet Sauvignon.

Malbec was raised out of obscurity by dedicated winemakers in Argentina to become a single varietal success story. In Bordeaux, it's called Cot, and was widely used for blending with Cabernet Sauvignon until it was gradually replaced by Merlot, which was less susceptible to late frosts and diseases. Under the name Auxerrois, it was once used to make the notorious "black wine" of Cahors, but that wine now contains up to 30 percent Merlot and other varieties. Malbec contributes less basic acidity to a blend than Merlot, but it can also provide distinct tannins and in France has been considered to add "rustic" elements to a wine. Wines made from Malbec typically have dark fruit flavors that vary somewhat according to region. In France, the wines are more likely to have a jammy blackberry taste, while those from Mendoza and other regions in Argentina have a more bountiful plum-like taste, which can include flavors like chocolate and anise. Malbecs are generally considered an excellent match for the grilled beef and pork that are the staples of the Argentine *asado*. As a result, the popularity of Argentine Malbec has spread rapidly to many steakhouses across the globe. No doubt this popularity will spark a renewed interest in the grape in Chile and Australia, where it has long been used for blending, as well as in other wine-growing regions.

Zinfandel can no longer claim to be the quintessential American grape, having been genetically identified as a sibling of **Primitivo,** which itself is a clone of the Croatian grape **Crljenak.** Like many other transplants, however, there is no doubt that it has thrived in California. There it makes generously alcoholic and tannic dry red wines with bold, brambly tastes replete of blackberries, black peppercorns and other fruits and spices, as well as hints of chocolate and aromas of violets and leather. Complex and layered, with ample alcohol to sustain its aromas, it makes great wines to noodle slowly through on a relaxed afternoon or evening. It is also used to make much sweeter and intensely flavorful, yet still refined, red wines, as well as cloyingly sweet "blush" rosé wines and a kind of port. In Italy, the wines made from the variety are characteristically drier and more bitter, but equally fruity, spicy and alcoholic.

Syrah or Shiraz, as it's known in much of the world, has a wonderful legend in which its origins are traced to a town named Shiraz in Iran, close to the area in which the earliest archeological records of wine cultivation have been found. Many have conjectured about whether the poet Omar Khayyám, when he lamented the absence of wine after death, was thinking of a Shiraz. A knight, the Chevalier de Sterimberg, was reported to have returned from the Crusades with some vines, become a hermit and built a chapel near the top of a hill, a hermitage, around which he tended his grapes. Today Hermitage, the town along the Rhône below the vineyard, is where the variety produces its most iconic wines. But the myth has been shattered in the cold, hard light of recent DNA tests. These show it to be a cross between two other varieties planted in the Rhône Valley by the Greeks long before the chevalier went off to the Crusades. Perhaps because of its homegrown origins, it has flourished in the northern valleys of the Rhône, where it's the dominant grape, although often blended with small amounts of other wines to soften it a bit. Like Cabernet Sauvignon and Nebbiolo, it takes time to ripen and its wines respond well to aging in wood. Dark, almost inky black, in color, dense, tannic and heavy with alcohol, its basic fruit taste of dark plums and black currants (cassis) lies tangled in tar and burnt rubber. These intense, deep flavors don't have quite the austere edges found in Cabernet Sauvignon and its brethren; instead it displays high alcohol content with an explosive, spicy, prickly, black-pepper quality. It can travel and is now a major variety in many of the warmer wine-growing regions, particularly in Australia, where it's deeply embedded in the culture. While beer may be a necessity, Shiraz is the secret ingredient for a great Australian barbie. In Australia, Syrah is sometimes blended with small amounts of Cabernet Sauvignon, as in the famous "Grange" produced by Penfolds. Although traditionally Australian Shirazes have exhibited rich, dark-berry and vanilla flavors, more recently, in cooler areas like Victoria, a lighter-colored, lighter-bodied style of Shiraz has emerged with a more raspberry taste. It is gaining in popularity in Argentina, where it's sometimes blended with Malbec and in South Africa, where some have cast it in the role of a savior for a wine industry that may not actually need saving, just a bit more political stability. The wines produced from Syrah in the northern Rhône tend to have more restrained fruit and exhibit elegant smoky elements, while the Australian and others tend to use a more fruit-forward style that is accented by a black-pepper spiciness.

Tempranillo, tough, leathery and smoky, is a variety every rancher should love. There is a quaint legend suggesting that it's a variant of Pinot Noir brought to Spain by pilgrims en route to Santiago de Compostela, but this too has been discounted by the DNA evidence. Despite being rather fragile, it is well traveled (under numerous aliases) and, despite its ability to withstand heat, it can perform well at high altitudes. In Spain, Tempranillo has traditionally been blended with

Garnacha and other varieties to make Rioja and other wines. Recently, there has been more interest in single varietal Tempranillo, both in Spain and elsewhere, and many excellent examples are available from the Ribera del Duero, Navarra and Penedès regions, where there is both sufficient altitude to maintain the vibrant tannins and an abundance of warm sun to thicken the skin and produce intense fruit flavors, reminiscent of cherries when young, and plums and darker berries as they age. In some Tempranillos, the texture and underlying fruit can suggest Pinot Noir (and/or Sangiovese), although with an overtone of tobacco, and sometimes vanilla and dark chocolate, the overall wine is much different. Like Syrah and Sangiovese, Tempranillo does not have the wild herbaceousness and ability to soak up tannin that Cabernet Sauvignon has (although some producers do try to force it). Consequently it tends to be softer and rounder and have an earlier drinking window. For this reason, Tempranillo is very versatile with food, and pairs well with a variety of grilled and roasted meats, poultry and fish. Its saltiness also makes it a good match for salty cheeses. Increasingly found on restaurant wine lists, it can be particularly useful when several people order different dishes.

Sweet Wine Varieties

Sémillon was once the most widely planted variety in South Africa, where wine drinkers have always had a notorious sweet tooth and the variety was called simply *Wyndruif* or "wine grape." During the nineteenth century, when sweet wines made regular appearances at the dinner table, it may have been the most widely planted variety in the world. The awe-inspiring wines, both sweet and dry, made from Sémillon in Bordeaux, particularly in the areas of Sauternes and Barsac, and in Australia's Hunter Valley and Adelaide Hills, demonstrate its extraordinary potential. What is produced in the rest of the world often seems rather dull and lifeless by comparison. If harvested early, Sémillon makes wines that are light yellow and brightly citric when young. With age and a bit of oak, the wines turn a deep golden color, gain a honeyed taste with hints of orange and acquire a stunningly rich and viscous taste. Great wines made from Sémillon are typically "botrytized" by allowing the ripe grapes to become infected by *Botrytis cinerea,* a mold otherwise known as "noble rot." *Botrytis* consumes water and shrivels the grapes, boosting acid and sugar levels, imparting a heady fragrance. Without the increase in acidity due to earlier harvesting, wines made from Sémillon have a tendency to seem rather lifeless, and are often blended with racier wines, like those made from Sauvignon Blanc, Muscadelle and even lean Chardonnays, to harden the edges and make them feel a bit crisper in the mouth. Many of the dry white wines in Bordeaux are made this way, as are some wines from Chile, California, Argentina and New Zealand. Many wines in these areas also use smaller amounts of Sémillon with reverse effect, to soften the edges of otherwise harsher wines. It's also used in some areas to make the extremely late-harvested ice wines and many Australians and South Africans like the mouth-filling, lemony flavors of wines made from ripe Sémillon grapes that are given a touch of oak.

Muscat is itself a family of varieties, whose colors range from golden yellow to green to black. Like the Pinots, they are prone to mutations that affect the skin color. Since the Muscat family also produces table grapes, it's perhaps not surprising that it's the variety most associated with a "grapey" taste, although its flavors can range from pears and apples to coffee and chocolate, depending on the specific variety and style. All three principal strains of the variety have an ancient pedigree and were spread by the Phoenicians, Greeks and Romans throughout the river valleys emptying into the Black Sea and the "White" (or Mediterranean) Sea, where they continue to be cultivated under a dizzying variety of names. Muscats are used to make everything from the sparkling light Astis of Italy and Alitas of Lithuania to the brandy-like Piscos of Chile and Peru and Metaxas of Greece. As fortified wines they are widely used in Spain and Portugal. A strain of Muscat is one of the three official grapes used in the production of sherry, while in Australia a strain known as "Orange Muscat" produces dessert wines with a decidedly orange aroma. Perhaps the most well known of the wines made from Muscat is the Muscat de Beaumes de Venice, first made famous through a positive review by Pliny the Elder in his *Naturalis historia*. For obvious reasons, it would be a mistake to think of this as a definitive exemplar of the variety, however. If you enjoy variety within a variety, Muscat is an excellent platform from which to launch an expedition into the more exotic varieties of wine.

Other sweet wines are made from the traditional red and white varieties listed above, most notably the Ausleses and "ice wines" made from Rieslings, the Molleaux wines from Chenin Blanc and the late-harvest Zinfandels. The higher sugar content in these wines will naturally produce a wine that is somewhat heavier in texture than their drier counterparts, but their basic fruit characteristics will usually be present.

Appendix C

Wine and Food Pairings

The following listing shows some pairings of foods with wines made from various grape varieties. The list is for you to scan, find foods you like and see what varietals show up with them the most. For each varietal and style, the wines I have in mind are those typical of the most well-known producing region: Burgundy for an old-world Pinot Noir or Napa Valley for a new-world Cabernet Sauvignon; Tuscany for an old-world Sangiovese or Mendoza for a new-world Malbec. These are, of course, very general guidelines and the success of the pairings will depend on the way the dish is prepared and the specific wine you choose. Quirks in these may interfere with the success of the match. The limitations will become obvious as you begin to experiment, but these pairings should provide a reasonably good place to start. Eventually, you'll want to move on to more specific matches as you find them.

Food	Varietal	Style
Meat-Centered Dishes		
Bacon	Gamay	New World
Barbecue Syrah (Shiraz)	New World	
Beef – ground (hamburgers)	Cabernet Sauvignon	New World
Beef – ground (frankfurters)	Merlot	
Beef – stewed	Pinot Noir	
Beef – roast beef	Pinot Noir	Old World
Beef – steaks	Cabernet Sauvignon	
Chicken – roasted	Chenin Blanc	
Chicken – fried	Chardonnay, Pinot Noir	New World
Duck	Pinot Noir, Merlot	
Ham	Almost anything	
Hamburger	Cabernet Sauvignon	
Kidneys	Merlot	
Lamb	Cabernet Sauvignon	
Liver	Sangiovese	
Pasta with meat and/or red sauces	Sangiovese	

Food	Varietal	Style
Pork chops	Riesling	
Pork – roasted	Cabernet Franc	
Pork – barbecued	Malbec	
Turkey	Almost anything	
Venison	Nebbiolo	
Seafood-Centered Dishes		
Anchovies	Garnacha	Rosé
Bluefish	Gewürztraminer	
Calamari	Gewürztraminer	Alsatian
Catfish	Pinot Grigio	
Ceviche	Sauvignon Blanc	New World
Crab	Chardonnay	
Dark, oily fish – *herring, mackerel, etc.*		
Grilled	Viognier	
Sauced - creamy	Chardonnay	Sparkling
Sauced – spicy	Roussanne	
Medium-colored oily fish – *char, pompano, salmon, tuna, etc.*		
Grilled	Pinot Noir	
Sauced – creamy	Pinot Noir	
Sauced – spicy	Syrah	
Firm whitefish – *halibut, Chilean sea bass, stripped bass, mahi-mahi, swordfish, etc.*		
Steamed	Syrah	Old World
Grilled	Pinot Noir	
Sauced	Barbera	
Flaky whitefish – *sole, flounder, etc.*		
Fried	Riesling	
Grilled	Chenin Blanc	
Sauced	Tempranillo	Old World
Lobster	Chardonnay	Old World
Mussels	Riesling	
Oysters	Muscadet	
Pasta with fish and/or white sauces	Pinot Gris	
Salmon	Chardonnay, Pinot Noir	New World
Scallops	Chardonnay	Old World

Food	Varietal	Style
Shellfish	Chardonnay	Old World
Shrimp	Viognier, Tempranillo	
Trout	Cabernet Franc	Old World
Tuna – fresh or roasted	Mourvedre	Rosé
Tuna – baked	Chardonnay, Pinot Noir	Old World

Fruit, Vegetable and Dairy Dishes

Food	Varietal	Style
Apples	Riesling	
Artichokes	Grüner Veltliner	
Asparagus – blanched	Riesling	Alsatian
Beans – black	Syrah	
Beans – green	Riesling, Merlot	
Beans – white	Sangiovese, Chardonnay	Old World
Broccoli	Chardonnay	New World
Broccoli rabe	Pinot Gris	Italian
Carrots	Sauvignon Blanc	New World
Chili peppers	Riesling	
Couscous	Syrah	Rosé
Corn	Chardonnay	New World
Curry	Chenin Blanc	
Eggplant	Cabernet Franc	
Eggs	Chardonnay, Riesling	Sparkling
Hummus	Pinot Gris	
Lentils	Pinot Noir	Old World
Mangoes	Riesling	Late-harvest
Melon	Chenin Blanc	Sparkling
Macaroni and cheese	Chardonnay	New World
Mushrooms	Pinot Noir	
Noodles – buttered	Nebbiolo	
Noodle soup	Chardonnay	New World
Onions	Pinot Gris	
Oranges	Riesling	
Pasta – plain	Barbera, Rosé	

Food	Varietal	Style
Pesto	Chardonnay	Old World
Potatoes – fried (plain)	Chardonnay	Sparkling
Potatoes – fried (with salt)	Tempranillo	
Potatoes – fried (with ketchup)	Sangiovese	
Potatoes – baked	Nebbiolo, Merlot	
Potatoes – roasted	Sangiovese	
Rice	Sake	
Risotto	Nebbiolo	
Salads – green or fruit	Chenin Blanc	
Salad greens – bitter	Sauvignon Blanc	
Salad greens – sweet	Chenin Blanc	
Soups – creamy / earthy	Barbera	
Soups – green vegetable	Grüner Veltliner	
Soups – tomato	Sangiovese	
Spinach	Chardonnay	Old World
Strawberries	Pinot Noir	Sparkling
Sweet potato	Chardonnay	New World
Tomatoes – fresh	Pinot Gris, Barbera	
Tomatoes – cooked	Sangiovese	
Desserts and Snacks		
Chili	Zinfandel	New World
Custard	Semillon	
Cookies	Muscat	
Pâté	Chenin Blanc, Riesling, Gewürztraminer	
Raspberries	Riesling	
Rice pudding	Muscat	Orange
Tandoori	Zinfandel	New World
Walnuts	Chardonnay, Syrah	Old World

Working with the pairings above should allow you to significantly improve your meals and your enjoyment of the wines you drink. You'll quickly notice that the way a dish is prepared or the style of the wine has a significant impact on the success of the pairing. With vegetable dishes, remember that raw vegetables tend to go better with white wines and red wines prefer their vegetables cooked.

In order to understand the heights to which food and wine pairings can reach, it's useful to experiment with some classic food and wine pairings. Here it's necessary to be a bit more specific about the wines and the way the food is prepared. If you find a match here that is accessible to you, you should try it. It would not be a classic unless most people found it seductively appealing.

CLASSIC FOOD AND WINE PAIRINGS

Food	Wine	Notes
Almonds	Manzanilla Sherry	Marcona almonds are best
Belon oysters	Muscadet	The tart, citrus vibrancy of the Muscadet resonates with the unusual metallic brininess of Belons
Camembert	Margaux	Use a well-aged Margaux for its salt-water finish
Cassoulet	Malbec	Both Malbec from Cahors and Cassoulet overwhelm most palates, but the combination is something different
Corn	Ribolla	Roast the corn
Corn chips	Muscadet	Serve with salsa
Chocolate cake	Banyuls (red)	Use a red, fortified Banyuls made from Garnacha (Grenache)
Foie gras	Sémillon	Use a botrytized Sémillon from Sauternes or Hunter Valley with lightly grilled foie gras
Graham crackers	Pinot Gris	Use a well-aged Alsatian Pinot Gris
Popcorn	Cava	Use a "Semi-seco" Cava that's well chilled to contrast with the heat of warm popcorn.
Prosciutto di Parma	Pinot Vert (Friuliano)	Use a Pinot Vert from Friuli-Venezia Giulia
Pork Roast	Côtes du Rhône	Prepare the roast in Provencal style with thyme
Tempura	Muscadet	Look for "Sur Lie" on the Muscadet label and use a traditional soy-based tempura sauce
Vanilla Ice Cream	Sherry	Use Pedro Ximénez Sherry
White Truffles	Barolo	Age unlocks the same spiced-earth feeling in the Barolo that there is in the truffles

A list of some basic wine and cheese pairings follows. Despite the general incompatibility between wine and cheese, the ultimate proof that wine's superiority as a beverage lies in its diversity is that there is a wine that will make a heavenly match with almost any cheese, of which there are, of course, thousands. The wine will not necessarily be enhanced, but the combinations should still work admirably. This listing is quite generic and is provided simply because the various pairings of cheese and wine can show just how subtle the pairings of food and wine can get.

If you're serious about cheeses, you'll often find a specific wine recommended when you read a description of a cheese. Be skeptical, however. Many of the recommended wines will work fine with the cheese, but are far from being the best choice. Sometimes, the cheese will benefit at the expense of the wine. Similarly, many wine producers, retailers and other food and wine professionals will recommend a cheese pairing for wines that seems less than optimal. Bear in mind that it's difficult to be an expert on both cheese and wine.

WINE AND CHEESE PAIRINGS

Varietal	Cheese
Cabernet Franc	Crumbly blue cheeses (and walnuts)
Cabernet Sauvignon	Salty cheeses like Cheddar and Danish Blue
Chardonnay	Soft, tangy cheeses like Brie and Colby
Garnacha	Light, nutty sheep's milk cheeses such as Idiazabal
Gewürztraminer	Intense cow's milk cheeses such as Muenster
Merlot	Hard cow's milk cheeses like Gruyere
Nebbiolo	Semisoft cow's milk cheeses like Swiss Fontina
Pinot Noir	Soft, rich aromatic cheeses like Époisses
Pinot Grigio	Semisoft cow's milk cheeses like Fontina Val d'Aosta
Port	Vegetarian blue cheeses, preferably Stilton
Riesling	Gouda, Edam or creamy, mild blues such as St. André
Sangiovese	Semisoft cheeses like Gorgonzola Piccante
Sauvignon Blanc	Light, creamy goat's milk cheeses such as Chèvre
Sémillon	Unpasteurized sheep's milk cheeses like Roquefort
Syrah	Spicy but mild goat cheeses such as Pave de Jadis
Tempranillo	Dry, mild cheeses like Manchego
Zinfandel	Sharp Cheddar or cheese flavored with peppercorns

Acknowledgments

This book wouldn't exist without the generous assistance and support I received from hundreds of people. Unfortunately, in the earliest stages, I didn't keep track of the many people who shared their frustrations with me or gave me advice about wine. Some were friends, but most were just people I met who had an interest in wine and a willingness to share it with a stranger. They may remember our discussion, but I either never knew their names or have forgotten them. I'm sorry I can't list them all here. I don't ever remember speaking to anyone who didn't advance the cause in one way or another.

More recently, I've been able to share my thoughts by giving copies of the manuscript of this book to various friends and acquaintances. They've also been remarkably generous with their time and support. George Vierra, a wine consultant and educator in Napa, shared notes and class outlines with me and helped me understand some of the technical details behind the excellent journal articles he has written for the wine trade. John Sharpe, former COO of Four Seasons Hotels and Resorts and trustee emeritus of the Culinary Institute of America, had a tremendous instinct for spotting what was missing and for giving me encouragement when needed. This book also reflects some of the philosophy and secrets shared with me by Neil McKensie and Alfredo Jara, of the Belle Haven Club. Ron Levine, M.D., as my personal physician, not only obliged me by reading the manuscript, but also by keeping me remarkably healthy through the many years while it was in the works. I was also fortunate to have the aid of Glen Silbert, M.D. and Gabrielle Bolton, M.D. who each provided me with valuable insights into the medical effects of alcohol. I am also grateful for the assistance that Charlotte Bartholomew gave me in producing the cover for the paperback version of this book. If there is technical merit in this book, it is largely through the interventions of these consummate professionals. Inevitably, it wasn't possible for even this battery of consummate professionals to catch all of my mistakes. The errors that remain are, of course, my own.

Several of my readers were themselves writers, writing coaches and editors. They were kind enough to take an interest, not only in wine, but in helping me become a better writer and provided me with valuable guidance and vital corrections of my grammatical and stylistic mistakes. I benefited tremendously from the generous assistance of Francis Furey and Emily Turner, both talented writers with a natural understanding of wine. Although Lindsey Reed could only squeeze in time to review the manuscript when she was in the passenger seat during a long road trip, she still provided me with some of the most valuable insights I received. It's easy to see why she's kept so busy as an editor. Bob Stiepock also coached me with the extraordinary patience that has endeared him to many students and other writers and my eagle-eyed (and formerly abstemious) copy editor, Angela Foote, not only added polish, but spared me from numerous embarrassing small mistakes.

Many others gave their time generously to this project, reviewing drafts and sharing their own experiences with me. They provided key insights, numerous corrections and essential moral support. I've listed them here in alphabetical order for want of any way to properly measure the relative value of their contributions: Dominique de Anfrasio, Peter Basilvesky, Tullio Borri, Nick Campbell, Mathew Clark, Kevin Craw, Richard Coppo, Katie Day Benvenuto, Marq and Mikiel de Bary, Matt DeFilippis, Charlie Degliomini, Bob Fein, Bob Friedman, Marty Gargano, Harriet Greenberg, Lindy Humphreys, Jim Kelsey, Bob Klingensmith, John Laxmi, Anna and Guy Longobardo, Joseph Matturro, Gerry Mintz, Scott and Johanna Moringiello, Rick and Stephanie Nathanson, Brett, Victor and David Nee, Vince (Jimmy) Orrico, Diane Reitano, Michael Remaley, Jim Shuman, Cynthia and Bill Sleight, Bob Singewald and Arnoldo Villafuerte. There are undoubtedly many more whom I have not properly recognized. I apologize for the oversight.

Index

heavy gravy, 130
herbal tastes, 95, 134, 179
herbs, 95, 127, 129, 134, 179, 184, 186
Hermitage, 99, 190
herring, 130, 194
Holy Grail, 167
Homer, 141, 166
honey, 128, 181
Howell Mountain district, Napa Valley, 189
horizontal tasting, 65
Hume, David, 103
Hungary, 181, 188
Hunter Valley region, Australia, 191, 197

I

importers, 109, 151, 171
iodine, 64, 127

J

Jayer, Henri, 104

K

Kabinett, 25, 181
Khayyám, Omar, 190
kiwi, 63

L

La Tâche, 54
labels, 26, 36, 43, 57, 92, 94, 120, 173, 197
labeling, 85-88
lactic acid, 90
Lafite-Rothschild, Château, 85, 88, 188
lamb, 120, 130
Latour, 188
Le Pin, 187
leathery taste, 64, 84, 190
Lebanon, 180, 185
legs, 45
lemons, 44, 60, 63, 89, 102, 127, 134, 147, 181
limes, 60, 63, 89, 102, 127, 181

location, 84, 86, 144
Loire Valley, 136, 180, 182, 186
longevity, 77, 79, 96, 167, 182
lower alcohol wines, 58, 123
luster, 45, 75, 145
lychee nuts, 182

M

mackerel, 127, 130, 194
Madeira, 175, 176
Maipo Valley, 189
Malbec, 55, 98, 149, 189, 190, 193, 194, 197
malic acid, 61, 63, 90
Margaret River, 189
Margaux, 188, 197
marmalade, 131
Marsanne, 183
matching, see pairing
Melon de Bourgogne, 183
melons, 62, 63, 180, 181
men, 106, 123, 143, 164
Mendoza, 189, 193
meniscus, 44
Merlot, 55, 98, 99, 128, 149, 178, 186, 187, 189, 193, 195, 196, 198
Michelin, Guide, 73
microclimate, 25, 83, 90, 97, 184
Middle Eastern cuisine, 22, 42
minerality, 14, 94, 96, 97, 102, 135, 179-181, 183
mint, 95, 134, 179, 188
Molleaux wine, 192
Montalcino, 98, 186
Montepulciano, 21, 98, 186
Morgon, 185
Morocco, 185
Mosel, 98, 120, 181
Mouton, 188
Mt. Veeder district, Napa Valley, 189
Müllerrebe, 183
Müller-Traube, 183
Muscat, 192, 196

Muskat-Silvaner, 180

N

Napa Valley, 51, 54, 98, 120, 150, 151, 180, 189, 193

Naturalis historia, 192

Navarra region, Spain, 185, 191

Nebbiolo, 98, 133, 187, 190, 194, 195, 196, 198

nerd, 158

new-world wines, 41, 42, 96, 98, 101, 136, 137, 185, 190

New Zealand, 41, 136, 180, 183, 184, 192

Newton, Isaac, 69

nobility, 145, 187

nose, 39, 46, 116, 156

note taking, 66

O

oak, 79, 96, 101, 150, 177, 188, 191

oily tastes, 95, 129, 130, 181, 183, 187, 190, 194

old-world wines, 41

olfactory epithelium, 39, 46

Oregon, 87, 181, 184

other drinks, 7, 24, 58, 76, 136, 163, 190

oxidation, 45, 90, 163, 174, 175, 176

oysters, 179, 183, 184, 197

P

pairing, 26, 27, 70, 75, 91, 102, 109, 119, 120-122, 125-139, 145, 181, 193, 196-198

palate, 10, 11, 18, 23, 29, 35, 39-42, 44, 47, 61, 67, 71-73, 100, 123, 124, 126-128, 130, 134, 136, 147, 148, 178, 188

Paracelsus, 166

Parker, Robert, 69, 71, 72, 150-152

Paso Robles region, California, 189

Pauillac, 88

peach, 180, 181

Penedès region, Spain, 189, 191

pepper, 44, 95, 133, 150, 187, 190, 195

Petit Verdot, 149, 150, 151

Petrus, 187

Peynaud, Emile, 166

phenols, 176

pickles, 127

Piedmont region, Italy, 187

pineapples, 44, 63, 102, 180

Pinot Grigio, 55, 89, 181, 194, 198

Pinot Gris, 181-183, 194-197

Pinot Meunier, 183

Pinot Noir, 47, 55, 98, 132, 133, 180, 183-185, 190, 193-196, 198

Pinot Vert, 197

Piscos, 192

Plato, 59

Pliny the Elder, 192

plum, 63, 179, 185, 187, 190, 191

Polpette alla Fiorentina, 75

Port, 198

ortugal, 94, 192

Pouilly-Fumé , 180

poultry, 129-131, 191

prices of wine, 105, 155

prices of wines, 5-8, 18, 19, 54, 70, 73-75, 77, 78, 81, 85, 107, 110, 141, 152, 173

Primitivo, *see Zinfandel*

Priorat, 185

procyanidins, 163

producers, 3, 7, 13, 20, 40, 44, 55, 57, 65, 71, 72, 78-80, 85, 87, 92, 93, 96, 98, 100, 104-106, 108, 110, 135, 141, 144-147, 150-152, 154, 171-173, 180-182, 184-187, 189, 191, 198

prohibition, 40, 55, 167

prune, 64

Prugnolo, 186

Puligny Montrachet, 120

Q

Spring Mountain district, Napa Valley, 189
Socrates, 166
soil, 13, 26, 54, 78, 83, 88, 90-92, 94, 96, 97, 100, 104, 184
sour taste, 58, 59, 60
South Africa, 41, 136, 180-182, 185, 190, 191
South America, 41
Spain, 87, 99, 185, 189, 190, 192
Spanna, *see Nebbiolo*
sparkling wines, 121, 180, 182
Spätlese, 25, 63, 120, 181
special occasions, 7, 48, 69, 75, 111, 113, 121, 122, 139, 155
spices, 44, 46, 95, 150, 185-187, 190, 191
spiciness, 5, 26, 39, 64, 123, 124, 182, 183, 188, 190, 194
spicy smell, 64
strawberries, 63, 185, 186
St. Émilion, 86, 186, 187
Steen, 182
Sterimberg, Chevalier de, 190
structure, 14, 20, 36, 54, 58, 59, 60-63, 66, 89, 90, 94, 97, 100, 132, 182, 183
styles of wine, 12, 14, 41, 42, 65, 74, 89, 92-94, 96-101, 108, 136, 170, 177, 179, 180, 182, 185, 186, 188, 190, 192, 193, 196, 197
sugar, 30, 41, 58, 59, 60-63, 78, 84, 107, 115, 133, 152, 181, 191, 192
sulfur, 90, 127, 163, 172, 173
Super-Tuscan, 21, 98, 188
sweet-sour taste, 22, 30, 31, 35, 42, 58, 60, 131, 132, 175
Sybil, 9
Syrah, 99, 133, 185, 190, 191, 193-196, 198

T

Taber, George, 55
tannic acid, 61, 79, 89, 90, 132, 133
tar, 95, 187, 190

tartaric acid, 59-61, 63, 89, 90, 132, 133, 186
taste buds, 35, 36, 39, 128, 132, 148
taste preferences, 38, 39, 40, 100
taste professionals, 37
temperature, 2, 8, 26, 28, 63, 79, 89, 106, 107, 111, 112, 116, 148, 157, 174, 179
Tempranillo, 99, 133, 185, 190, 194, 195, 196, 198
terroir, 83, 97, 104, 108
texture, 19, 30, 37, 38, 57, 58, 61, 64, 66, 89, 90, 95, 97, 101, 109, 125-127, 129, 130-133, 138, 139, 179, 191, 192
thirst, 5, 165, 166, 179
tobacco, 95, 187, 191
tongue, 3, 9, 29, 35, 36, 39, 44, 46, 48, 59, 60, 61, 133, 148
Traminer, 182
turnips, 127
Tuscany, 21, 100, 186, 189, 193
Tyrene, 175

U

University of California, 138

V

value, 5, 6, 15, 18, 19, 33, 53, 55, 73, 75, 78-81, 107, 149, 153, 200
vanilla, 44, 46, 95, 185, 186, 190, 191
varietal characteristics, 92, 98
varietals, see grape varieties
variety, 7, 8, 14, 21, 25, 30, 32, 34, 38, 41, 46, 51-53, 56, 64, 87, 89, 91-93, 98, 99, 101, 102, 108, 134, 144, 148, 150, 170, 177-186, 190-192
veal, 130, 186
vegetable dishes, 130, 196
vegetable flavors, 10, 44, 95, 127, 129, 179, 188
vegetable tastes, 95, 187, 191
vertical tasting, 65
Victoria region, Australia, 190
vinegar, 5, 45, 59, 89, 127, 176

vinegar taste, 127, 174, 176

vineyards, 2, 26, 42, 54, 78, 80, 84, 85, 86-88, 95, 100, 103, 104, 106, 107, 144-146, 170, 171, 184, 188, 190

vintage, 33, 65, 71, 73, 79, 83, 97, 103-107, 109, 115, 144, 145, 151, 175

Viognier, 55, 183, 194, 195

vitamin C, 89, 161

viticultural areas, 86

vodka, 60

Volnay, 184

Vosne-Romanée, 184

Vouvray, 182

W

warm climate, 45, 123, 179, 185

Webster, Daniel, 156

weight, 12, 35, 37, 41, 57, 58, 123, 126, 129, 130, 131, 162

white wine, 12, 18, 30, 44, 55, 62-64, 89, 90, 94, 95, 99, 114, 127, 128, 138, 177, 178, 181, 184, 191, 196

Willamette Valley, Oregon, 181

wine and cheese, 128, 129, 197

wine experts, 2, 3, 20, 32, 36, 37, 102, 148

wine lists, 6, 7, 74-76, 80, 86, 113, 122, 142, 143, 157, 191

wine media, 53, 55, 56, 67, 124, 141, 146, 147, 153, 161

wine tastings, 7, 144

Wine Spectator, 54, 149-151

winemakers, 41, 89, 94, 141

women, 36, 123, 164

wood, 46, 79, 95, 97, 108, 179, 190

woodland tastes, 95, 188

Wyndruif, 191

Y

young wine, 61, 115

Z

Zinfandel, 55, 189, 196, 198

17159427R00114

Made in the USA
Charleston, SC
29 January 2013